Caring for Hindu Patients

Edited by

DIVIASH THAKRAR
General Practitioner, Northwood
GP with Specialist Interest in Cardiology, Hillingdon Hospital

RASAMANDALA DAS
Educational Consultant based in Oxford
specialising in Education and Hinduism

and

AZIZ SHEIKH
Professor of Primary Care Research and Development
University of Edinburgh

Foreword by
DR SAM EVERINGTON OBE
General Practioner, Tower Hamlets

Radcliffe Publishing
Oxford • New York

Radcliffe Publishing Ltd
18 Marcham Road
Abingdon
Oxon OX14 1AA
United Kingdom

www.radcliffe-oxford.com
Electronic catalogue and worldwide online ordering facility.

British Library Cataloguing in Publication Data

A catalogue record for this book is available from the British Library.

ISBN-13: 978 185775 598 5

Typeset by Pindar New Zealand (Egan Reid), Auckland, New Zealand
Printed and bound by Hobbs the Printers, Southampton, Hampshire, UK

Contents

Foreword

Mahatma Gandhi's life is an inspiration to all of us. He was a great healer of individuals and communities. Learning about his religion and way of life helps us as health professionals to be far more than scientists. To be really successful, we have to use our role to help individual patients with all their health needs, while at the same time improve the health of all the communities in which we live. Many of us were trained to be scientists. Today with the access to knowledge that most people have, and a more equal society, we need to have far more inclusive and adaptable skills. The relationships we have with our patients need to range from being a scientist to a counsellor, from a friend to a partner in self care. Our knowledge also needs to be much wider. To improve the health of our patients, we need to be able to address all the issues which affect their health and wellbeing. This includes not only diseases but also their environment, education, employment and spiritual health. To be successful, we need to know far more about the context of people's lives, their religions and the cultures in which they have been brought up.

This book is vital to any modern-day health professional. It helps us diagnose and care for Hindu patients, approximately one in a hundred of our community, but goes beyond this on a journey that makes us far better health carers. It teaches us to speak the 'language' of all our patients. If we learn to do this, any consultation will have a better outcome. In particular, the 80% which are about long-term illness. Evidence now suggests that some of the biggest improvements in the care of chronic disease will come from helping our patients to manage their own illnesses. For us to make all this happen, we have to understand the context in which all our patients live.

Dr Sam Everington Barrister, OBE
General Practitioner, Tower Hamlets
Deputy Chair, BMA, 2004–07 (Acting Chair, 2007)
Ministerial Advisory Board on Primary Care (Access), 2007–present
May 2008

This is a concise and easy to read text which provides valuable information for the busy medical professional working in a modern multi-cultural practice. This book is a goldmine of insights into Hinduism with helpful summaries and appendices on matters as they relate to health. Understanding culture and tradition improves the care and communication we have with our patients and this book covers many of the important issues and rituals from birth through to death. There are also clear signposts to other resources and key sites on the web. This book should be available in every healthcare environment.

DR IVAN F TROTMAN MD FRCP
Consultant Physician, Mount Vernon Hospital
Clinical Director, Mount Vernon Cancer Network

How does one rise to the challenge of representing the multiple facets and interpretations encapsulated within Hinduism for those interested in caring for the Hindu patient? This concise book rises to this challenge and elegantly succeeds by approaching the subject matter innovatively by focusing on the key concepts that explain both the similarities and differences between different Hindus. Through the metaphorical cycle of birth, marriage and death, the authors guide the reader towards developing cultural sensitivity to aid their consultations as well as inform them of Hindu beliefs and practices relevant to the care of the Hindu patient. The case studies and the appendices full of practical tips are a great help to busy practitioners faced with Hindu patients on a regular basis.

DR SABBY KANT MRCGP
GP and Medical Author

The Hindu faith is considered 'a way of life' pervading all aspects of its adherents' day-to-day existence. As a Minister of the Hindu Faith and medical doctor I consider this book a comprehensive and exceptional account of Hindu ethos coupled with clear practical applications when interacting with Hindu patients.

DR RAJ PANDIT SHARMA
President, Hindu Priest Association UK

Preface

Providing high-quality clinical care for the diverse communities that now make up British society is an important challenge for the NHS; furthermore, the extent to which this is achieved is a clear indicator of our social commitment to equal opportunities. However, achieving this aspiration is no easy task, as evidenced by persistent health inequalities – and this despite the good intentions of the skilled and diligent professionals who plan, deliver and evaluate care. Many people from within these minority faith and ethnic communities believe that this, to a large extent, reflects an inadequate understanding of the relationship between religious and ethnic identities, and the impact of these identities on access to care and the quality of its delivery.

There is now a large and relatively well-established Hindu community in Britain, members of which are making a substantial and important contribution to the social, economic and intellectual development of these isles. This contribution is increasingly recognised. Far less appreciated is that members of this same community have particular health and social care needs.

Caring for Hindu Patients is an extremely welcome publication. For the first time, it provides carefully considered, evidence-based and readily accessible insight into the healthcare needs of British Hindus. With its contributions from well-respected members of the British Hindu community and others, it will, we hope, prove to be a much-valued resource for medical, nursing and other healthcare professionals, working both in hospitals and community settings.

We wish this landmark work the success it deserves.

> **National Council of Hindu Temples,**
> **Hindu Forum of Britain,**
> **Hindu Council UK,**
> **BAPS Swaminarayan Sanstha and ISKCON**
> *May 2008*

Contributors

Vipin Aery
Ex-Co-Temple President, ISKCON Ujjain
Ex-General Secretary to the National Council of Hindu Temples (UK)

Dr Roger Ballard
Anthropologist
Director, Centre for Applied South Asian Studies, University of Manchester

Aude Cholet
Advanced Community Specialist Dietitian and Community Dietetics Services
  Manager, Northwick Park Hospital

Rasamandala Das
Educational Consultant based in Oxford and specialising in education and
  Hinduism

Krishna Dharma
Writer and broadcaster

Dr Nilamani Gor
General Practitioner

Dr Bhavesh Kataria
General Practitioner, King's Langley

Dr Paul Oliver
General Practitioner, Peacock Surgery, Nottingham
GP Tutor, Division of Primary Care, University of Nottingham Medical School

Dr Heenakumari Ghanshyambhai Patel
General Practitioner, Peacock Surgery, Nottingham
Teaching Fellow, Division of Primary Care, University of Nottingham Medical
  School

Dr Bhanu Ram
Resident in Internal Medicine and Primary Care
William Beaumont Hospital, Royal Oak, Michigan, USA

Dr Vibha Ruparelia
Consultant Obstetrician
The Whittington Hospital, Highgate, London

Professor Aziz Sheikh
Professor of Primary Care Research and Development
Division of Community Health Sciences (GP Section)
University of Edinburgh

Nima Suchak
Freelance journalist

Dr Diviash Thakrar
General Practitioner, Northwood
GP with Specialist Interest in Cardiology, Hillingdon Hospital

Acknowledgements

But those who always worship Me with exclusive devotion, meditating on
My transcendental form – to them I carry what they lack, and I preserve
what they have.

Bhagavad-Gita 9.22

We take great pleasure in expressing our gratitude to the book's contributors,
especially the authors who generously donated time from their busy schedules;
first to write articles and then to respond to the numerous (and sometimes
conflicting) requests for revision.

Our specific thanks go to members of the publishing team at Radcliffe
Publishing, who have been helpful, patient and supportive, even in the face of
delay. Thanks also to our spiritual guides and mentors, especially Srutidharma
Das, Raju Mehta and Kripamoya Das. For academic input, thank you to Surinder
Shandilya, our Sanskrit expert, and to Paramtattvadas Sadhu and Yogivevekdas
Sadhu for their spiritual insight and diligent proofreading.

Numerous well-wishers have graciously helped by reviewing successive draft
chapters; they include Dr Richard Grocot-Mason, Dr Simon Dubrey, Reverend
Bruce Driver, Mr Om Prakash Sharma, Dr Rohit Barot, Dr Bhan, Pat Bacon and
Dr Raj Pandit Sharma. Many thanks to you all! And special thanks to Vinay Tanna
and Prasant Kotecha, who helped with introductions to different people.

Our gratitude to Dr Sam Everington, who kindly wrote the foreword, and to
the diverse Hindu organisations whose representatives worked collaboratively
to make this a joint effort, and to show that we can indeed be inclusive, despite
personal, philosophical and theological differences.

We also wish to thank our families, who were patient with us and provided
much-needed support.

Finally, our thanks to you, the reader, for taking an interest. We hope that this
book proves an invaluable addition to your library and assists you in the laudable
and painstaking task of delivering sensitive and impeccable healthcare.

Diviash Thakrar, Rasamandala Das and Aziz Sheikh
May 2008

Introduction

We live in an increasingly diverse society, in which ethnicity and religious affiliation are two key dimensions of personal identity. Within the UK, the growing Hindu community is estimated at well over half a million, of whom approximately one third are born and raised in Britain. Overall, Hindus have integrated well into British society, enriching its cultural life in the fields of the arts, commerce, education and professional practice. However, social diversity presents a number of interesting and complex challenges. One arena in which issues and misunderstanding arise is the sometimes emotionally charged area of delivering and receiving healthcare. This book aims to enhance the practitioner's awareness of issues pertinent to the care of Hindus, and to provide insight into how services may be provided sensitively, with respect for Hindu values, practices and worldviews.

There is now a welcome burgeoning body of literature on caring for people from specific ethnic and faith cultures. Therefore, one may be forgiven for asking, 'Why should we add a further publication?' There are two main reasons: first, although many generic accounts of Hinduism are available, they are neither professionally accessible nor clinically relevant; and, second, attempts till now have typically represented 'outsider' accounts, which – even with best intentions – fail to grasp and communicate the real spirit of Hindu belief and practice.

In an attempt to overcome these limitations, we have deliberately invited contributions from authors who are not only professionals but are either practising Hindus or intimately linked to the community. Our selection of authors and editors also reflects the long-standing plural, multicultural and multi-religious nature of Indian society. Of the three editors, one is a practising Hindu of white, European stock (Rasamandala Das), and the other two are of South Asian origin: one a devout Muslim (Aziz Sheikh), the other a practising Hindu (Diviash Thakrar).

The book itself is divided into two main parts. The first (Chapters 1 and 2) explores the origins of the tradition, tracing the historical development of philosophy and practice, and the migration trends underpinning the emergence of the UK community; this part includes a summary of current demographic data on British Hindus. The second part (Chapters 3 to 6) examines the practical issues relevant to the delivery and reception of care and – in some cases – issues of compliance. Topics discussed include dress, diet, communication, birth customs, the extended family, contraception, abortion and terminal care. The remainder of the book includes a useful glossary, and appendices covering the various deities and Hindu festivals, principal Hindu organisations, guidance on useful websites, and appropriate diet sheets.

This book is by no means comprehensive; it cannot entirely accommodate the diversity of Hindu belief and practice, nor adequately address the tensions between long-standing religious ideals and contemporary practice. However, despite these limitations, we anticipate that this publication will be a useful addition to the libraries of healthcare professionals. We also hope that it encourages readers to further explore the rich, spiritual culture of Hinduism.

Diviash Thakrar, Rasamandala Das and Aziz Sheikh
May 2008

PART ONE

The Hindu tradition

CHAPTER 1

Hinduism: the tradition speaks for itself

Vipin Aery, Rasamandala Das and Krishna Dharma

In this opening chapter, our authors provide a concise and cohesive overview of Hinduism. After examining the challenges in precisely defining the tradition, and its diverse and evolving strands, they explore certain recurring features and unifying themes. They particularly focus on the Hindu worldview, its philosophical underpinnings, and its outward expression, consisting of both spiritual practices and their broader, social dimensions.

Introduction

Dating back at least 5000 years, Hinduism is the oldest of all religions,[1] and yet endures today as a healthy, colourful and exuberant tradition. It has clear connections to India, where it remains the majority religion, but its social, spiritual, cultural and linguistic influences now visibly extend across the globe.[2] It also has important links to other 'Eastern religions', including Jainism, Buddhism and Sikhism.

However, it is difficult to determine how Hinduism started. Unlike most other religions, it has no single founder, no one scripture, no commonly agreed set of teachings and no unified code of conduct. Throughout its extensive history, there have been hundreds of key figures, teaching various philosophies, writing thousands of holy books, and modelling diverse practices. This inescapable diversity makes Hinduism particularly hard to define. Nonetheless, there are clearly some 'common elements and unifying themes'.[3] In an attempt to more suitably define Hinduism, it is often referred to as 'a way of life' or 'a family of religions'.[4]

Defining Hinduism

Scholars suggest that the term 'Hindu' was first coined by 8th-century Persians to refer to people on the far side of the River Indus (at the time called the River Sindhu). Its original meaning was not specifically religious but cultural, political and geographical. Practitioners adopted the term only around the 15th and 16th centuries, feeling obliged to differentiate themselves from followers of other, often hostile faiths. The noun 'Hinduism' was only coined around the 19th century, and is now widely accepted. Despite this, its precise definition remains somewhat arbitrary and the subject of extensive debate.[5] Whichever definition we choose, we are likely to find exceptions.

Some adherents claim that one is 'born a Hindu', but there are now many Hindus of non-Indian descent. Texts often imply that all Hindus believe in an impersonal supreme entity, but important strands have long venerated a personal God. Outsiders often deride Hinduism for its polytheism, but many adherents claim they are monotheists (though in a more inclusive way than their Abrahamic counterparts). Some Hindus define orthodoxy as compliance with the teachings of the Vedic holy texts (the four Vedas and their supplements). However, still others identify their tradition with *Sanatana Dharma*, the universal religion that transcends any specific body of sacred literature. Western authors often draw inordinate attention to the caste system, but many Hindus consider such practices mere social phenomena or, more often, as an aberration of their original social system, called *varnashrama*. Nor can we resort to defining Hinduism according to belief (a term Hindus little use), for not all subscribe to the same key concepts, such as *karma* and reincarnation.

Although it is not easy to define Hinduism, we can say with certainty that it is closely connected to India, its culture and its sacred texts – but it also extends beyond them.

Sanatana Dharma

The tradition itself has attempted self-definition based on adherence to certain holy books, the *Vedas* and their supplements. Veda is a Sanskrit word meaning 'knowledge'. Apparently, this universal wisdom was first passed down orally and only later committed to writing. Most Hindu traditions date this to about 5000 years ago. Scholars, particularly those from the West, often believe the texts to be more recent, dating the compilation of the first book, the *Rig Veda*, to around 1000 BC.

Significantly, the Vedas themselves do not include the terms 'Hindu' and 'Hinduism'. Rather, they discuss 'Sanatana Dharma'. Sanatana means eternal and dharma loosely translates as 'religious law' or 'religious duty'. More precisely, it means 'that which sustains us according to our inner nature'.[6] Hindus often prefer to call their tradition Sanatana Dharma, meaning 'the eternal religion'. This name implies that the tradition is timeless, teaching truths (such as the existence of the eternal soul) relevant to all people, at all times, in all places. The eternal nature of the living entity is considered to be engagement in the service of God. The teachings endeavour to bring the living entity back on this path. With this understanding, Hindus tend to regard their path as inclusive. Indeed, most Hindus do not reject other authentic religions, believing them to be but different paths towards the same divinity.

The historical development of Hinduism

Hinduism's early history is the subject of much debate, for three main reasons.[7] Firstly, there are differences of opinion between more traditional Hindus and many Western scholars. Secondly, Hinduism is not really a single religion, but embraces many quite autonomous strands. Thirdly, Hinduism has no precise starting point. It goes back at least 5000 years and maybe much further (with some believers claiming that it is eternal!).[8] Hinduism therefore has a long and complex history. To study Hinduism thoroughly it is essential to also consider its own worldview.

Hindus believe that time is cyclical and eternal, rather than linear and bounded. Even the universe (or universes) are repeatedly created and destroyed. Time moves in cycles, much like the four seasons. Texts define four successive ages (*yugas*), designated respectively as golden, silver, copper and iron. Apparently, during the golden age, people were all pious and religious. With each successive age, good qualities diminished, until we reached the current iron age, marked by cruelty, hypocrisy and materialism.

More recent history is traced back 5000 years to the beginning of the current *Kali Yuga*, an era extensively described in the Hindu epic, the *Mahabharata*. It was at this time that Lord Krishna, widely believed to be God himself, appeared on earth and spoke the Bhagavad-Gita, now one of the most important philosophical texts.

Many scholars, however, have a rather different view of Indian history. Following in the footsteps of early Indologists, such as Max Muller, some still teach that Hinduism originated outside of India, and was brought to the sub-continent by a race called the Aryans, who conquered the Indus Valley around 1500 BC. The religion of the Aryans blended with that of the indigenous Dravidians (who now live in South India), laying the foundations for what we now call Hinduism. However, this is contested by different parties, some trying to prove an origin that supports the supremacy of their own culture. Hence, some Hindus claim that India was the cradle of civilisation,[9] countering the colonial interpretation that the highly civilised forms of early Hinduism could only have come from Europe. Such claims often draw on recent archaeological evidence from the Indus and Sarasvati valleys. Despite extensive debates, it is unlikely that anyone will conclusively establish the exact history of the tradition.

Hindu teachings

Hinduism has neither a common doctrine nor a single scripture. It places more emphasis on orthopraxy (correct practice) than orthodoxy (correct belief), encouraging freedom of thought within relatively stringent codes of moral and spiritual conduct. More than the Abrahamic traditions, it succeeds in combining religion with philosophy,[10] and faith commitment with reflective search for truth. It does not generally exhort followers to declare allegiance to a single faith, belief or creed.

However, despite a relatively inclusive approach, Hinduism has distanced itself from doctrines that reject its scriptural authority; for example, Jainism and Buddhism. Within the orthodox systems, there are six main schools or, more precisely, *darshanas* ('ways of seeing'). The most popular perspective today is called *Vedanta*, meaning 'the culmination of all knowledge'. In typical Hindu style, Vedanta philosophy does not entirely reject the other darshanas but has attempted to assimilate and explain them.

Although Hinduism encourages flexibility of thought, some concepts are almost universally accepted. They contribute to the distinctive character of Hinduism, and lend unity to its diverse strands. Below is an overview of Hindu thought, with the main concepts highlighted in bold.

An overview of Hindu theology[11]

> Almost all Hindus believe that the real self (**atman**) is eternal, made of spirit (**brahman**). The atman (or soul) sometimes takes on a temporary material covering (physical body) and, by identifying with matter (**prakriti**), is entrapped by illusion (**maya**). Impelled by lust, greed and anger, he endures the cycle of repeated birth and death (**samsara**). Each atman creates its unique destiny determined by the universal **law of karma** (action and reaction). Under the influence of **eternal time** and the three material **gunas** (qualities), he moves throughout the **creation**, sometimes reaching higher planets, sometimes moving in human society, and at other times descending into lower species. Human life gives opportunity to achieve **moksha**, liberation from this perpetual cycle, through re-identifying with the eternal Supreme (brahman). Hinduism accepts **different paths towards this common goal** (union with the Supreme). At the same time, it stresses adherence to universal principles through performance of one's specified duty (**dharma**), as revealed through authorised **holy books** and the authentic **guru** (spiritual mentor).

Most Hindu theology is discussed in relationship to three main concepts or 'truths', and the respective relationships between them. They are (1) the self, (2) matter and (3) God. It is in discussing the third item that Hindu traditions exhibit great diversity, and many debates centre of the precise conceptual relationship between the Supreme and the individual soul.

What is significant is that Hindu thought usually begins with discussing the self (which is somewhat known) before examining the nature of subjects more remote, such as the Supreme. In other words, Hindu epistemology suggests that without comprehension of the real self, as spirit, it is difficult to apprehend God with any cognitive clarity.

1 The atman (real self)

The atman ('real self') resides in all living creatures, as the source of life and awareness. Hindu theology refutes the ideas that consciousness emerges from a mature combination of matter, or that transient combinations can ever produce an enduring self. Although bodily designations (male or female, white or black) are false, superfluous to the true self, the common perception of continuing identity implies the presence of a real, enduring self.[12]

Western philosophy generally discerns mind from matter.[13] Distinctively, Hindu thought holds that spirit (brahman) is different from both gross matter (the physical body) and its subtler forms (e.g. mind). This conclusion may be reached through a comparative analysis of spirit and matter. Reflection on spirit (the self) reveals that it is unchanging (hence eternal) whereas matter (mind and body) is ever-changing (hence temporary). The self is active and conscious; matter is inert and unconscious. Ironically, the presence of the soul within the body misleads us into considering matter itself the source of life, a view often thrown into turmoil by terminal disease, death and other traumatic events.

> 'As the embodied soul continuously passes, in this body, from boyhood to youth to old age, the soul similarly passes into another body at death. A sober person is not bewildered by such a change.'[14]

> 'Those who are seers of the truth have concluded that of the nonexistent [the material body] there is no endurance and of the eternal [the soul] there is no change. This they have concluded by studying the nature of both.'[15]

Hindu belief in an eternal, uncreated self lays foundations for a complete world-view, and further concepts that explain pre-existence, destiny and 'the problem of evil'. 'Karma' is a multi-layered term that simultaneously refers to action, the corresponding reactions and the accumulated stock of such reactions. It is free will and individual karma that determines the transmigration of the atman from one body to another, a process commonly called reincarnation. Good karma, based on noble aspirations, results in an elevated existence on higher planes. Conversely, bad karma impels the soul to fulfil base desires within lower species. Although God awards all living beings the appropriate results of their behaviour, each soul is entirely responsible for his or her own destiny. Such destiny is formulated only while invested with the responsibility of human life. Animals suffer karma but do not create it.

'As a person puts on new garments, giving up the old ones, the soul similarly accepts new material bodies giving up the old and useless ones.'[16]

'In proportion to the extent of one's religious or irreligious actions in this life, one must enjoy or suffer the corresponding reactions of his karma in the next.'[17]

The human form of life is also special for the opportunity to escape the cycle of birth and death. The aspiration for liberation suggests that Hindus view life in this world (but not life itself)[18] as an undesirable situation, beset by the miseries of birth, disease, old age and death. However, birth as a human is considered most fortunate, provided one makes use of its rare facilities and to become free from the dictates of matter.

2 Matter
Matter (prakriti) refers to the non-conscious elements of God's creation, including the physical body and the mind. Matter is transient, undergoing the three stages of creation, maintenance and destruction. These relate to three respective qualities or 'modes' (or, in Sanskrit, 'guna'). There are three gunas: goodness (*sattva*), which sustains; passion (*rajas*), required for creation; and ignorance (*tamas*), responsible for all forms of decay and destruction. The notion of the three gunas is central to lifestyle choice, making moral decisions, and the Indian system of medicine called *Ayurveda*. The three gunas, and their respective functions, also correspond to the three main deities (as described below).

3 God
Most of the theological differences in Hinduism focus on two questions, namely: (1) the nature of God and (2) the identity of God. With regard for God's nature, the various schools tend to give different emphasis to three main aspects of the Supreme, called *brahman, antaryami*[19] and *bhagavan.*[20]
1 Brahman refers to conscious spirit, the all pervading aspect of God (God everywhere).
2 Antaryami refers to the super-self, within the heart of living beings (God within).
3 Bhagavan refers to the personal form of God (God outside, or beyond this world).

'That brahman is in front and in the back, in the north, south, east and west and is also overhead and below. In other words, that supreme brahman effulgence spreads throughout the material and spiritual skies.'[21]

'The Supreme Lord is situated in everyone's heart, and is directing the wandering of all living beings.'[22]

'Bhagavan is [defined as] he who possesses, without limit, the six types of opulence – strength, fame, wealth, knowledge, beauty and renunciation.'[23]

Theological debates similarly address the relationship between God and the self. The two wings of that debate are represented by the monists and the dualists. Other schools of thought either qualify one of these perspectives or attempt, in different ways, to synthesise the two.

Monists stress the pre-eminence of the brahman (all-pervading) aspect of God. They consider the atman to be identical with God in all respects. The aim of liberation is to become one with brahman (God as an impersonal force). The practitioner strives to realise that he or she is God.

Dualism stresses the personal form of God as bhagavan. He is eternally distinct from the soul, and has a spiritual form with limitless qualities. The worshipper's aim is to become the eternal servant of the Supreme, who has intrinsic form, activity and personality.

Monism and dualism both reconcile the acceptance of many deities with belief in one God. For monists, the various gods and goddesses are equal and represent different attributes of a single, impersonal Supreme. The dualistic schools[24] are more accurately designated as 'monotheistic'; that is, they believe in a single god who is intrinsically a person. However, their stance is better described as 'inclusive monotheism',[25] for it not only affirms the truth of a single, personal God but simultaneously the existence of numerous lesser deities, often allocating them different hierarchical positions.

> 'The portrayal of Hinduism as entirely or largely polytheistic is wrong. Even the claim that all Hindus believe in one God as an impersonal energy (brahman) is misleading. I was born into a prominent tradition that holds that God is ultimately a person, and that Krishna and Vishnu are higher than other deities.'
>
> *Dr AB Patel*

Most Hindu traditions also respect the notion of antaryami, or 'the Lord within', though he is given particular importance by those who follow the path of meditation.

Most Hindus also believe that God is both male and female, usually through the notion of 'divine couples'.[26] There are three main deities, called the *Trimurti*, each of whom has a wife or consort, as shown in Table 1.1.

The main branches of Hinduism not only debate the nature of the Supreme but are defined by their particular focus of worship. We should note that the three main traditions do not correlate to the Trimurti. The main focuses of worship include two of the Trimurti, namely Vishnu (2) and Shiva (3). To these two, Shakti (6) is added, though many of her devotees also venerate the other two goddesses, Sarasvati (4) and Lakshmi (5). Apparently, due to a curse from his wife, Brahma (1) is not widely venerated.

The three resultant traditions are called *Vaishnavas, Shaivas* and *Shaktas*. It is important to note that:

1 Vaishnavas often worship Vishnu though one of his forms, such as Krishna and Rama, whom they consider two of his 10 main incarnations.[27]
2 Followers of Shiva, called Shaivas, often consider their chosen deity to be supreme and therefore also responsible for creation and sustenance.
3 Shakti, venerated by Shaktas, has many other names, such as *Durga, Parvati*, and *Mataji* (respected mother).
4 There is a further, fourth denomination, the *Smarta* tradition, whose members worship five main deities.

TABLE 1.1 The main deities and their wives

THE TRIMURTI	THE WIVES OF THE TRIMURTI
1 Brahma, the creator	4 Sarasvati, the Goddess of Learning and the Arts
2 Vishnu, the sustainer	5 Lakshmi, the Goddess of Wealth and Good Fortune
3 Shiva, the destroyer	6 Shakti, the personification of Mother Nature

The other important deities are almost always related to the above-mentioned six. For a more complete list, *see* Appendix 1. We should also note that many Hindus do not confine themselves to any one tradition, and are happy to worship a number of deities. Additionally, some do not subscribe to any of the four main strands. These include members of the 19th century 'reform movements', such as the Arya Samaj, whose members venerate a formless spiritual entity.

Sources of authority

Hindu teachings are derived from two principal sources: the Hindu sacred literature (the Vedas and their corollaries); and the corresponding realisations of holy people, especially gurus (spiritual teachers). There is also a third authoritative voice, namely 'God within'. He is called the *antaryami* (the witness to all our acts) and the *caitya guru* (the 'hidden guru'). Hinduism promotes self-autonomy to the degree that a person acts according to divine instruction – and 'the conscience' – rather than worldly compulsion.

Hindu wisdom was first transmitted orally and only later written down, usually in Sanskrit. In South India, the Tamil language is also held in high esteem, and even considered sacred, much like Sanskrit in the north. More recent texts are written in vernacular languages, including Hindi, Punjabi, Bengali and Gujarati. The main texts are classified into two main sections, the *shruti* ('that which is heard') and the *smriti* ('that which is remembered').

TABLE 1.2 Main Hindu texts

MAIN SHRUTI TEXTS	MAIN SMRITI TEXTS
The Four Vedas:	The Vedanta Sutra (codes of philosophy)
1 Rig Veda	The Itihasas ('Histories' or 'Epics')
2 Yajur Veda	(a) the Ramayana (b) the Mahabharata
3 Sama Veda	The Bhagavad-Gita (part of the Mahabharata)
4 Atharva Veda	The Puranas (stories)
The 108 Upanishads (philosophical texts)	The Dharma Shastra (law books, e.g. the 'Manu Smriti')

Most traditions teach that assimilation and application of knowledge are dependent on having an authentic spiritual teacher. To be authorised, a guru should normally come in an unbroken line of teachers, known as a *sampradaya*. These sacred lineages often trace their origins to a divine source, such as an incarnation of the Supreme. The genuine guru is expected to be spiritually knowledgeable, detached from material enjoyment, and fully devoted to God.

> 'Just try to learn the truth by approaching a spiritual master. Inquire from him submissively and render service unto him. The self-realised souls can impart knowledge unto you because they have seen the truth.'[28]

Spiritual practices

For Hindus, spiritual activities are usually executed as part of one of four main *margs* (paths) or '*yogas*', which practitioners may choose according to their disposition and level of spiritual advancement. These four main disciplines are:
1 Karma-yoga: the path of selfless action.
2 Jnana-yoga: the path of knowledge.
3 Raja-yoga (or astanga-yoga); the path of meditation.
4 Bhakti yoga: the path of devotion.

Most popular in contemporary Britain is bhakti-yoga.[29] What most people call 'yoga' is actually *hatha yoga*, a preliminary step on the path of meditation; its purpose therefore goes beyond health and physical well being. In fact, all the above 'yogas' ultimately aim at self-realisation and union with God, as indicated by the literal meaning of the term yoga, 'to join', from which we derive the English word 'yoke'.

Some Hindu teachers list 'five activities considered essential for any practising Hindu' as follows:
1 worship
2 festivals
3 pilgrimage

4   rites of passage
5   dharma (executing one's socio-religious obligations).

1 Worship

Worship in Hinduism is very broad, and may include many apparently cultural or artistic facets, such as dance and drama. The following table lists 10 main forms of worship, though many can be subsumed under '*puja*'.

TABLE 1.3 Ten types of worship

Meditation/Japa/Prayer – individual and internal practices.
Puja – ritual worship, especially of the deity. It often includes:
Arti – the greeting ceremony, offering lamps, incense, etc.
Bhajana or Kirtana – hymns and chants.
Darshana – taking audience with the deity (or holy person).
Prasada – offering and respecting sacred food.
Parikrama/Pradakshina – circumambulation (e.g. of the deity).
Seva – active service (to the deity, holy people, etc.).
Pravachana – talk or lecture on the scriptures, often philosophical.
Havana – the ancient, sacred fire ceremony (as during rites of passage).

The most important categories are (1) meditational practices, and (2) puja (ritual worship).

Meditational practices

Perhaps the most popular form of meditation is japa. It involves the quiet or silent recitation of a mantra, a string of sacred syllables such as the Hare Krishna mantra or 'Om Namo Shivaya'. It is generally performed on a *mala*, a string of 108 prayer beads made from tulasi wood for Vaishnavas, or *rudraksha* berries for Shaivas. Another popular and traditional form of meditation is the recitation of the Gayatri mantra. It is traditionally observed by *brahmins* (members of the priestly class) at dawn, noon and dusk, using the sacred thread wrapped around the thumb of the right hand.

Japa and other forms of meditation are considered to purify the heart of materialistic desires, promote self-realisation, and invoke a natural affinity for God. The prayer beads and sacred thread are usually treated with great respect. Some practitioners will use additional, visual aids to meditation, such as pictures of their chosen deity. Although listening to sacred songs and chants or religious talks are listed (above) as separate forms of worship, they are also considered meditative practices, helping to fix the mind on God.

Puja

Puja means worship, and particularly refers to the daily, ritualistic adoration of the murti (sacred image) within the temple. It involves the bathing and dressing of the deity and the offering of various auspicious items, such as water, perfume and flowers. The worship culminates in the offering of food, followed immediately by the most popular ceremony, called *arti*, in which lamps and other auspicious articles are again offered as an act of devotion, and then shared with the congregation.

An important and ubiquitous feature of Hindu life is worship at the home shrine, usually organised by the womenfolk. Domestic puja is usually a scaled-down version of the grand temple services. It may only be offered daily or even once a week, unlike the scheduled temple worship, which must continue from early morning until late evening.

Worship of the sacred image (murti)

In Hinduism, the temple (*mandir*) is considered the home of God, or the particular deity residing there. The sacred image, fashioned from marble, metal or wood, should be made in strict accordance with directions found in Vedic texts. The resultant form, known as the murti, is ceremoniously installed in the temple and worshipped with great pomp and devotion.

Worship of the sacred image is one of the most misunderstood aspects of modern Hinduism.[30] Vedic theology accepts that God is within everything, and the deity especially represents him. Hindus are enjoined to worship only authorised and properly installed deity forms, and through prescribed methods. This is distinct from unauthorised worship (or 'idol worship'), in which an imaginary form may be capriciously constructed and worshipped.[31]

> Visitors to Hindu temples will often notice both male and female forms on the shrine. Hinduism acknowledges both male and female aspects of the Supreme. The female aspect is the eternal consort of the Lord, and is described as the supreme energy (shakti) of God, who is the supreme energetic. They are thus inseparable and equally important. Some examples of these divine couples are Krishna (male) and Radha (female), and Rama (male) and Sita (female).
>
> *Dr Sailesh Patel*

2 Festivals

The Hindu year is punctuated by many opportunities to celebrate.[32] Festivities usually commemorate important events in the life of a saint or a particular Hindu deity; for example, *Janmastami*, marking the birth of Krishna. Additionally, there are seasonal festivals, such as *Holi* (the spring festival of colours), and events celebrating family ties, such as *raksha bhandan* when girls tie amulets on their brothers' wrists.

Diwali, falling in October or November and coinciding with the New Year for most Hindus, is most widely celebrated. The dates for this 'festival of lights' and most other holy days are calculated using a lunar-solar calendar and vary annually according to the Gregorian calendar. A list of festivals and approximate dates can be found in Appendix 2.

Festivals are times for celebration and remembrance, focusing on spiritual matters and bringing together friends, families and communities. Main practices include fasting and feasting, the distribution of sacred food (*prasada*), giving in charity, attending the temple and visiting relatives. Festivities also include all forms of decoration, traditionally using fruits, leaves, flowers and other gifts of nature.

3 Pilgrimage

The importance of pilgrimage in Hinduism is demonstrated by the continuing popularity of the *Kumbha Mela* festival, the largest human gathering in the world. Hindus abroad have also developed local pilgrimage sites, such as their favourite temples. Nonetheless, India remains a special place and many British Hindus combine pilgrimage with visits to relatives. Pilgrimage is especially important for those retiring from householder life, and is performed largely for purification and gaining spiritual merit. It may involve performance of religious rites, such as the scattering of ashes or the offering of sanctified food (*shraddha*) for the family's deceased. Other activities include taking *darshana* (audience) of specific deities, circumambulation and the observance of vows and austerities, such as celibacy and walking barefoot to respect sacred ground. The most famous pilgrimage town is Varanasi on the River Ganges.

4 Rites of passage

Hindu rites of passage are not just formalities or social observances, but serve to purify the soul at critical junctures in life. The word *samskara* means 'mental impression', and its observance is intended to create a favourable mentality, suitably concluding one phase of life and positively starting the next.

Although some traditions mention 10 rites of passage, or up to 16 (and occasionally even more), four are currently popular,[33] namely:
1 *Jatakarma* – birth ceremonies (plus a few others in childhood).
2 *Upanayana* – initiation (the sacred-thread ceremony).
3 *Vivaha* – the marriage ceremony.
4 *Antyeshti* – funeral and rites for the dead.

These ceremonies, often accompanied by a *havana* (sacred fire ceremony), are further explored in Chapters 4 and 6.

5 Dharma and social observances: the family

The notion of dharma (religious or righteous duty) extends the ideals of spiritual progress to the arena of social life. Traditionally, the basic building block of Hindu society was the joint or extended family, consisting of three or four generations living together. Men and women had distinct duties. The women collectively shared domestic responsibilities, and males provided the income for the family. Elders often took important decisions. Within the family, property usually passed from father to son, and men took many of the decisions, though older women carried considerable influence. When women married, they usually joined their husband's family.

Hindu families still demonstrate relatively firm ties of affection. Scripture has elaborately defined the dynamics of the various family relationships, and relatives are given specific terms of address and endearment, unlike the practice of designating all as 'aunt' or 'uncle'. For example, in Hindi, the paternal grandfather and grandmother are addressed as 'Dada' and 'Dadi' respectively; on the maternal side they are called 'Nana' and 'Nani'.[34] Often the suffix 'ji' is added to these terms to convey respect (e.g. Dada-ji).

The extended family traditionally provides shelter and support for the elderly, the disabled and the less economically able. Children are expected to show gratitude to parents by supporting them in retirement and old age. An important aspect of Hindu family life is the interdependence between members. Marriage itself is viewed as a broad socio-religious commitment, rather than a partnership between individuals. The extended family can often provide considerable practical and emotional support, as for example when children are born.

Despite this, social trends indicate that the extended family is becoming less popular, especially outside India. Young couples often value the freedom that the nuclear family offers. They often shun arranged or assisted marriages and, naturally, are also adopting other aspects of a Western lifestyle.

Varnashrama and caste

In modern times, Hinduism's reputation for inclusivity has been tarnished by the caste system, which allocates members to a particular social class (*varna*) and occupational subclass (*jati*). Caste practice has spawned all manner of social abuse, particularly of the 'untouchables' (also called 'the scheduled castes'). Since Indian independence, measures to address these anomalies, such as the reservation of governmental jobs and university placements, have been implemented. Some Hindus claim that this apparent solution contradicts traditional notions of meritocracy, specifically by denying places to more qualified candidates. Nonetheless, with improved education and financial stability, caste discrimination appears to be diminishing.

Despite changes, certain communities, including many prevalent in the West, still encourage endogamy or associations based on common social, regional and ideological values (not dissimilar to some Western clubs and institutions). Most noticeably, some parents still insist that their children marry within the same *jati*.

Caste practices are not peculiar to Hinduism. They are found within other faith communities (though the community may not endorse them), including Islam, Christianity and Sikhism, both within and beyond the Indian subcontinent. Consequently, some Hindus attempt to explain caste as a sociological phenomenon, entirely distinct from religious principles. However, this argument is challenged by explicit mention of the four *varnas* within the most ancient of Hindu religious texts, the Rig Veda.[35]

To accommodate this, many Hindu thinkers consider modern practices an aberration of that original system. That older system, going by the name *varnashrama-dharma*, allocated individual duties according to four *varnas* (broad social classes) and four *ashramas* (stages in life). Scriptural examples of people changing *varna* suggest that it permitted social mobility. Apparently, the system later became hereditary, reserving prestigious jobs for those born in higher *varnas*, and disadvantaging members of the lower classes, particularly the untouchables, who have been collectively (and perhaps erroneously) called 'the fifth varna'. Mahatma Gandhi supported the untouchables, whom he renamed *Harijans* (children of God). Many reformers now use Gandhi's teachings and example to argue against both caste and *varnashrama*, which they wrongly conflate. Gandhi himself recognised the difference between varnashrama-dharma (which he supported) and the hereditary caste system (which he vehemently opposed).

> *Varna* is generally determined by birth, but can be retained only by observing its obligations. One born of the brahmin parent will be called a brahmin, but if he fails to reveal the attributes of a brahmin when he comes of age, he cannot be called a brahmin. He would have fallen from brahmin-hood. On the other hand, one who is born not a brahmin but reveals the attributes of a brahmin will be regarded as a brahmin.
>
> *MK Gandhi*[36]

The four varnas were primarily a means towards social organisation, ensuring that all found fulfilment though careers and livelihood consistent with their talent and disposition. Ashrama means 'place of spiritual shelter' or 'hermitage', indicating that all four stages of life are meant for the cultivation of spiritual life. The four varnas and four ashramas are shown opposite.

The social dimensions of Hinduism have undergone significant changes throughout history. During Muslim domination (*c.* 1200–1750 AD), there arose many bhakti (devotional) traditions, which opposed the rigid caste system and propounded a spiritual egalitarianism. These gave rise to many of the contemporary forms of Hindu devotion. During the British administration (from about 1757 onwards), the influence of Western thought spawned many reform movements, which later helped India towards independence and planted seeds for later forms of Hindu nationalism. It was also during the time of the British Raj that significant migration from India began to affect the global landscape of Hinduism, eventually bringing many Hindus and their religion and culture to the shores of Britain.

TABLE 1.4 Varnas and ashramas

FOUR VARNAS	FOUR ASHRAMAS
Brahmins – priests, teachers and scholars	Brahmachari ashram – celibate student life
Kshatriyas – government, police and armed forces	Grihastha ashram – married life
	Vanaprastha ashram – retired life
Vaishyas – farmers, traders and business people	Sannyasa ashram – renounced life
Shudras – artisans, craftsmen and workers	

Migration to Britain

Major migration began in the 19th century, when Hindus sought employment – mainly as indentured labourers – in places such as Fiji, Mauritius, the Caribbean, Central America, and South and East Africa. From the 1960s many others migrated, especially to the UK (mainly from East Africa) and to Canada and the United States (mainly from India itself). There are now large communities of Hindus worldwide, especially in Europe and North America. There are also large communities in Bali, Nepal, Trinidad and Sri Lanka. India itself is home to many religions, but today over 80% of its people are Hindus.[37]

Major migration to the UK is relatively recent. Hindus started arriving in significant numbers shortly after the Second World War. However, the main wave of immigration, from East Africa, spanned the sixties and early seventies. They largely settled in inner-city areas, and were often relatively poor, many having lost their wealth upon expulsion from Uganda. They became menial workers or started small businesses as grocers, newsagents and clothing manufacturers. The natural centres for these fledgling communities were the first austere temples converted from old buildings such as church halls. However, by the close of the 20th century, the Hindu community had become socially and economically well established, as evidenced by academic results, business achievement and an increasing number of costly and prestigious temples.

Main groups represented in contemporary Britain

Although early temples were relatively eclectic, drawing from a number of traditions, later complexes are often denominationally based, representing specific transnational movements with their respective spiritual leaders (gurus). Those well established in Britain include the BAPS Swaminarayan Sanstha, ISKCON (the Hare Krishna Movement), the Ramakrishna Mission and the

Pushti Marg community. There are numerous yoga and meditation groups and other organisations, such as the Satya Sai Baba Foundation, which do not classify themselves as Hindu.[38]. There are also many local community groups, often based on jati (occupationally based social groups) and several national umbrella organisations, such as the National Council for Hindu Temples, the Hindu Council UK and the Hindu Forum of Britain. For more details of these groups, *see* Appendix 3.

Conclusion

This essay is a concise introduction to the great traditions collectively known as Hinduism. The vast canon of Vedic writings contains teachings on all areas of human endeavour, many of which are being rediscovered and used in Western society today. For example, the medical teachings known as Ayurveda are increasingly popular, as are the texts on sacred space known as Vastu (the Indian version of feng shui). Practices such as yoga and meditation also stem from Vedic teachings and are firmly integrated in our lifestyles.

Perhaps the main contribution of Hinduism, in the authors' view, lies in its teachings on spirituality, as found in texts such as the Bhagavad-Gita. With their instructions on how to nurture inner peace, inclusivity and spiritual happiness, these texts have over the years found many adherents from the West. Whether or not members of the medical profession share any personal interest in Hinduism, or in broad spirituality, they are sure to meet many Hindus. We hope that this chapter will help them to better understand this rich and ancient tradition, and at least give some understanding on the background to Hindu values, customs and culture as encountered in the healthcare environment.

Key points

- Hinduism started at least 5000 years ago and may be much older.
- The word 'Hindu' was perhaps first given by the Persians about 1100 years ago to refer to the inhabitants beyond the Indus River. The word was adopted by insiders much later and the term 'Hinduism' only emerged in the 19th century.
- Many practitioners prefer the term Sanatana Dharma, meaning 'the eternal religion'.
- Hinduism isn't a single religion, particularly not in terms of belief. Rather, it is often described as 'a way of life' or 'a family of religions'.
- There are certain concepts accepted by most Hindus. This includes belief in an eternal self that transmigrates according to the law of karma. The goal of most Hindus is moksha, liberation from this perpetual cycle.
- In a broad sense, the Hindu tradition encompasses a range of approaches to God, from overt polytheism to strict monotheism. The majority believes in one God, either as monists (believing in an impersonal, all-pervading energy)

or as monotheists (believing in one Supreme God, usually with many lesser deities).

◈ The acceptance of a spiritual teacher (guru) and accepting initiation are important elements in the Hindu tradition.

◈ The worship of the sacred image (murti) is central to much Hindu practice.

◈ There are numerous Hindu festivals, usually involving fasting, feasting and other observances. Perhaps the most popular in Britain is Diwali, the festival of lights.

◈ Many British Hindus still go on pilgrimage, particularly to India and often in conjunction with visiting relatives.

◈ The modern caste system is most likely an aberration of the original social order called varnashrama, which divides society into four classes and human life into four stages.

◈ There are four main traditions: Vaishnavas (who worship Vishnu), Shaivas (who worship Shiva); Shaktas (who worship Shakti); and Smartas (who worship five deities).

References and notes

1 Klostermaier K. *Hinduism: a short introduction to the major sources.* Oxford: Oneworld Publications; 2000. p. 1.

2 Flood G. *An Introduction to Hinduism.* Cambridge: Cambridge University Press; 1996. p. 1.

3 Ibid.

4 Knott K. *A Very Short Introduction to Hinduism.* Oxford: Oxford University Press; 1998. p. 112. Knott states that this term was coined by the modern Hindu philosopher Sarvepalli Radhakrishnan.

5 There are entire books written on the subject. For example, *see* Llewellyn JE, editor. *Defining Hinduism: a reader.* London: Equinox; 2005.

6 Das R. *The Heart of Hinduism: a comprehensive guide for teachers and other professionals.* Aldenham: ISKCON Educational Services; 2002. p. 24.

7 Das R. *21st Century Religions: Hinduism.* London: Hodder Wayland; 2005. p. 6.

8 Johnsen L. *The Complete Idiot's Guide to Hinduism.* Indianapolis: Alpha; 2002. p. 1.

9 Das R. *Atlas of World Faiths: Hinduism.* London: Franklin Watts; 2007. p. 9.

10 Klostermaier K. *A Concise Encyclopedia of Hinduism.* Oxford: Oneworld Publications; 1998. p. 12.

11 Lipner J. *The Face of Truth.* Basingstoke: The Macmillan Press; 1986. p. ix. Lipner attempts to disabuse the idea that Hinduism is entirely philosophical rather than theological. It's also worthy to note that, at the time of writing, Oxford University includes courses in 'Hindu Theology' in connection with the Oxford Centre for Hindu Studies. This overview has been adapted from: Das R. *The Heart of Hinduism,* op. cit., p. 6.

12 Without the notion of a continuing self, many commonly held notions relating to kinship, life-management or criminal justice become meaningless. Although the sense of identity with the body is false, the perceived but distorted idea of continuity affirms rather than negates the existence of a self.

13 Honderich T, editor. *The Oxford Companion to Philosophy*. Oxford: Oxford University Press; 2005. p. 221.

14 Bhaktivedanta Swami AC. *The Bhagavad-Gita As It Is*. Los Angeles: Bhaktivedanta Book Trust; 1989. Verse 2.13.

15 Ibid., verse 2.16.

16 Ibid.

17 Bhaktivedanta Swami AC. *The Srimad Bhagavatam*. Los Angeles: Bhaktivedanta Book Trust; 1987. Verse 6.1.45.

18 Many writers make this illogical assumption.

19 Or sometimes 'paramatman' (the supreme self); however, some traditions use paramatman to refer to the supreme soul of the universe, rather than the Lord in the heart.

20 Or 'Ishvara'.

21 Das R. *The Heart of Hinduism*, op. cit., p. 20. The three aspects of God, as given here, are said by Vedic texts to be simply different realisations of one truth. An analogy is given of seeing a hill from a distance, where it appears like a cloud. Upon closer inspection one sees that it is a hill, and when seen even closer one can see a village on its side with buildings and people. God is said to be realised gradually in the same way, from brahman, the all pervading energy, to bhagavan, the Supreme Person.

22 Bhaktivedanta Swami AC. *The Bhagavad-Gita As It Is*, op. cit., verse 18.61.

23 Das R. *Vaishnava Verse Book: a compendium of Vedic verse*. Borehamwood: Bhaktivedanta Books Ltd; 1990. p. 282.

24 That is, those who are purely dualistic (the followers of Madhva) and those who accommodate some form of qualified dualism, usually by acceptance of some elements of monism.

25 Lipner J. *Hindus: their religious beliefs and practices*. London: Routledge; 1994.

26 Rather than hermaphrodites, although there are examples of this.

27 Some traditions consider Krishna to be Supreme, even higher than Vishnu.

28 Goswami, S. *Readings in Vedic Literature: the tradition speaks for itself*. Los Angeles: Bhaktivedanta Book Trust; 1990. p. 93.

29 It often accommodates elements of the other paths.

30 Rosen S. *Introduction to the World's Major Religions: Hinduism*. London: Greenwood Press; 2006. p. 83.

31 For an example of a thorough exposition on the science of worship of the murti, *see* Valpey KR *Attending Krishna's Image: Chaitanya Vaishnava Murti-seva as devotional truth*. London: Routledge; 2006.

32 Jackson R and Nesbitt E. *Hindu Children in Britain*. Stoke-on-Trent: Trentham; 1993. p. 75.

33 Klostermaier K, op. cit., p. 163.

34 Das R. *The Heart of Hinduism*, op. cit., p. 106.

35 Specifically in the hymn called the Purusha-shukta. Other writers also suggest that varnashrama is integral to Hinduism. For example, *see* Rosen S, op. cit., p. 11.

36 Gandhi MK. In search of the Supreme. *Harijan*. 1934; 28 September: 260. It should be self-evident that a person is not necessarily going to be the same as his or her parents. For example, a son of a lawyer may have no inclinations or abilities for that profession, whereas the son of a manual labourer could rise to become a high court judge. There

is some evidence that this type of social mobility was originally accommodated within ancient Indian society, and was at least held as an ideal.

37 Das R. *21st Century Religions*, op. cit., p. 5.
38 Often because they are concerned about the sectarian nature of the very term 'Hinduism', as opposed to other, more inclusive nomenclatures such as 'Sanatana Dharma'.

CHAPTER 2

Social and demographic characteristics of Britain's Hindu population

Dr Roger Ballard

In this chapter, Dr Ballard introduces us to the demographic diversity within the British Hindu community. He opens by explaining the origins of the country's Hindu population, and the various trajectories of migration. He further explores the challenges faced by Hindus living in a foreign culture, and notes their resilience, resourcefulness and socioeconomic achievement. He concludes by looking to the future, touching on possible implications for healthcare professions.

Introduction

Since the end of the Second World War, Britain's Hindu population – then no more than a few thousand – has grown rapidly. In the 2001 census, when respondents were first asked to specify their religious affiliation, 557,985 residents identified themselves as Hindu. Of these, just over one third were British born. However, while the ancestral origins of virtually all of Britain's Hindus lay in the Indian subcontinent, not all came directly from India. A substantial proportion belonged to families whose members had previously settled in Britain's overseas colonies – especially those in East Africa – from where they subsequently moved to the UK.

This chapter explores the origins of Britain's Hindu population, the way in which its members established themselves in a largely unfamiliar sociocultural environment, and the largely successful, and increasingly varied, trajectories of adaptation for both settlers and their locally born offspring. In so doing, this chapter also seeks to highlight some of the most significant sources of internal differentiation within the diverse British Hindu population.

Origins and settlement patterns
Pioneers of the Hindu presence in the UK

Hindu visitors began arriving in Britain at the start of the 19th century. Among the earliest arrivals were sailors recruited to serve on East Indiamen making the long return journey to London from Indian ports such as Bombay, Madras and Calcutta. Soon afterwards, educated young men made their way to Britain to obtain professional qualifications, especially in law and medicine. The same ships carried representatives of major Indian business houses, seeking to base themselves in London and Manchester, and spendthrift maharajahs keen to splash out on the delights and extravagancies of Edwardian Europe. Later, the First World War saw the arrival of numerous units of the Indian army bound for the French battlefront; a process repeated two decades later during the course of the Second World War.[1]

Until the 1940s, only a tiny minority of Hindus took up permanent residence in the UK. Most stayed for a few years, returning home upon completion of their business. However, dramatic changes occurred after the end of the war. Not only did India gain independence, but Britain's manpower planning went amiss. As the post-war boom took off, acute shortages of labour compelled Britain to look to its former colonies to fill the emerging deficiencies. The most acute demand lay in the industrial sector, where hot, dirty and ill-paid jobs in foundries and textile mills were virtually unfillable. Similar gaps emerged further up the labour market. For example, the newly created National Health Service, and the lack of local professional training, precipitated a sharp increase in demand for nurses and doctors. In the absence of adequate numbers of locally trained professionals, the Health Service had little alternative but to recruit from overseas.

However, few South Asian migrants to Britain were directly recruited by prospective employers. Most made their own way to Britain, and only subsequently found work though a process of chain migration, in which friends, relatives and class-fellows of earlier pioneers followed in their predecessors' footsteps. As a result, settlers in the UK did not come from across the length and breadth of the subcontinent: instead, the majority arrived in concentrated streams from specific communities and localities within two broad regions: (1) the Punjab, deep in the interior north-west of Delhi, and (2) the western seaboard state of Gujarat, north of Bombay.

Migration to East Africa

Emigration from Gujarat was a function of the region's long-standing transnational connections across the Indian Ocean. Gujarat's many creeks and rivers were ideal sites for boat building, and for three millennia provided safe harbours for local merchants trading with Mesopotamia, Red Sea ports and the east coast of Africa. For most of this period, Gujaratis merely set up temporary overseas trading posts. However, when the British took control of Kenya and Uganda towards the end of the 19th century, and subsequently of Tanganyika after the First World War, many Gujarati settlers began to cross the Indian Ocean, taking advantage of new commercial opportunities opened by British entrepreneurs pressing into the African interior. As merchants expanded their businesses, thousands of Gujaratis, largely from peasant-farming families, migrated to East Africa to open inland trading centres. Here, even in the remotest villages, such *dukanwalas* (storekeepers) became a familiar sight.

Migrants were also needed to build and operate the East African railways; for these purposes, skilled craftsmen were recruited from the Punjab as well as Gujarat, and largely from communities whose hereditary occupations were as masons, carpenters and blacksmiths. Like the dukanwalas, many of the most successful came from the Lohana community, whose ancestral occupation was as traders and merchants.

The social order of colonial East Africa was strictly hierarchical. At the top, British settlers formed a highly privileged elite, whose members routinely reserved for themselves the most fertile land and prestigious jobs. At the bottom, in a position of subordination, were members of the indigenous African majority. This left the 'East African Asians' (as South Asian settlers were called) to form what can best be described as 'the filling in the colonial sandwich'. Although firmly excluded from the colonial elite, by dint of hard work and imaginative deployment of entrepreneurial resources, the East African Asians swiftly lifted themselves clear of the bottom of the pile. Largely as a result of their efforts throughout the first half of the 20th century, the local economy grew rapidly, attracting a steady inflow of further settlers from South Asia, especially Gujarat and the Punjab. As these settlers grew prosperous, their lifestyles became increasingly westernised, at least in material terms. However, given their systematic exclusion by members of the European elite, East African Asians turned to each other for mutual support, creating their own colonial structures based on their own distinctive social, cultural, religious, linguistic and familial conventions. Hence, just as East Africa's white settlers reconstructed a comprehensively English world around themselves, so each of the many components of the East African Asian population set about constructing their own equally distinctively structured ethnic colonies in what was becoming an ever more overtly plural East African social order.[2]

During the course of the 1960s, all this came to an end. As Britain reluctantly granted independence to its East African colonies, Asian settlers found themselves caught in a vice. Despite their subordination to the European elite, most had been sufficiently successful to occupy positions of substantial privilege over the indigenous population. Immediately after independence, South Asians not only dominated commercial enterprise but filled the majority of professional and managerial roles within government and administration. In other words, they occupied precisely the socioeconomic slots into which Africans expected and aspired to move. The resultant moves towards Africanisation – reaching its peak in 1972 with Idi Amin's expulsion of 70,000 Asians from Uganda – led to a steady outflow of Asian settlers. While some returned to India, many more sought alternative destinations in Canada, the United States and Britain.[3]

The consolidation of the South Asian presence in Britain

Up to 1962, migrants from South Asia could freely enter Britain. As Commonwealth citizens, the moment they stepped ashore they gained rights and privileges identical to other British subjects, and could stay indefinitely. However, as the inflow from the subcontinent steadily increased, so did popular alarm about the consequences. From 1962, draconian measures were introduced in an effort to control the inflow of 'New Commonwealth' citizens (as those of non-European descent were euphemistically described).

With new measures slow to take effect, demands to control the inflow became increasingly clamorous. Consequently, restrictions became ever tighter, and were eventually extended to include 'non-patrial' British passport holders, a category deliberately constructed to include (and, hence, exclude) East African Asians. These measures eventually took effect: the inflow of people of colour into the UK was undoubtedly much less than it might have otherwise been. Nevertheless, the 1960s and 1970s comprised the peak period of South Asian migration into the UK, either directly from South Asia, or more indirectly from the many colonial territories from which Britain was withdrawing. Besides the East African colonies, these included Fiji, Singapore, Mauritius and many Caribbean islands. Since the late 1970s, immigration from these sources has steadily declined. The more recent inflow comprise both highly qualified professionals (such as doctors and information technologists) and spouses or prospective spouses of British-born Hindus. Thus far, those from India who have contracted such transnational marriages have almost invariably taken up residence in Britain. However, as India grows more prosperous, there are sound reasons to anticipate significant migration in the reverse direction.[4]

Demography

Although post-war immigration greatly enhanced the diversity of British society, only much later were these developments formally recognised. It was not until 1991 that an 'ethnic question' was introduced into the national census. The introduction of a question identifying religious affiliation had to wait until the following census in 2001. At long last, this made it possible for social scientists to construct a numerically accurate picture of Britain's new-found condition of ethnic, racial and religious plurality.

Age pyramid

During the early stages of settlement, migrant populations usually contained a disproportionate number of males, and people in their twenties and thirties (since young adult males exhibit a relatively strong propensity to move overseas, leaving their families to later catch up with them). However, as Figure 2.1 demonstrates, by 2001 Britain's Hindu population had reached a condition of relative maturity, in which the process of family reunion was virtually complete: men only marginally outnumbered women. Nevertheless, the shape of the pyramid still provides clear evidence of this group's migrant origin. The population size tails off sharply for those over the age of 50: not so much the result of higher rates of mortality, but of far fewer older members migrating to Britain.

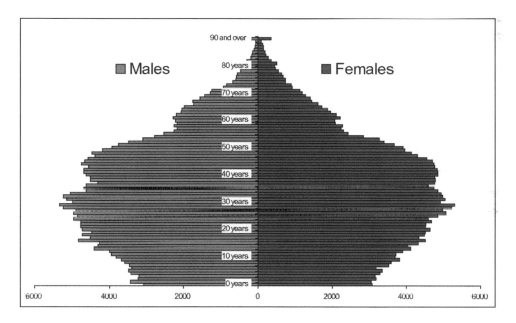

FIGURE 2.1 Age distribution of the Hindu population of England and Wales, 2001

Next to this, the most significant feature of Figure 2.1 is the way in which the pyramid diminishes towards the bottom. The youngest cohorts are little more than half the size of those around the age of 30. This suggests that, in common with many other affluent and upwardly mobile, contemporary populations, the fertility rate among Britain's young Hindus has fallen sharply, and is currently running at substantially less than replacement rate.

Meanwhile, from a medical perspective, there are also significant developments at the other end of the age spectrum. Although this population is relatively mature, it nevertheless includes a disproportionately low numbers of retirees. The pyramid in the diagram is but a snapshot in time: all the bars in Figure 2.1 move upwards, one step each year (though they will diminish somewhat due to increased mortality rates). Hence the proportion of elderly people in the Hindu community is set to rise very sharply in the years to come, imposing a sharply increased level of demand on corresponding services. Planners should urgently take note of the warnings inherent in these statistics.

Household and family composition

In addition to providing data about individuals, the census data also allows us exploration of the size and shape of Hindu households. As Figure 2.2 shows, the current pattern of Hindu household structures differs markedly from that within the UK population as a whole.

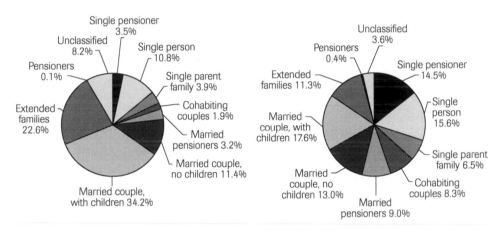

FIGURE 2.2 Hindu household structures (a) as compared with those in the UK population as a whole (b)

In making sense of these differences, the patterns revealed by Figure 2.1 also need to be kept in mind. For example, the current relative paucity of elderly people among British Hindus partially accounts for, in Figure 2.2(a), much smaller-sized segments for both single and married pensioners. However, the most striking way in which Hindu household structures differ from others is the sharply increased salience of both extended families (those with three or more adult members), and households in which dependent children live with their parents. The result is that the proportion of single person households, single parent households and those in which the parents merely cohabit (rather than being formally married) is sharply reduced. Hence, the least one can say about Britain's Hindu population is that it is strongly family oriented, and that family breakdown is relatively rare.

Hindu commitment to the maintenance of tight-knit networks of kinship reciprocity, and to active community construction within the context of their many jati (subcastes or kinship groups) has had positive socioeconomic consequences. The census confirms that although many settlers arrived in Britain with next to nothing, and took jobs in which few others were interested, they and their

British-born offspring have achieved a remarkable degree of prosperity. Indeed, in comparison with the indigenous majority, they are now moving into a position of relative socioeconomic advantage.

Diversity

Careful attention must also be paid to not only the mean achievements of any given population but also the diversity found within it. Diversity in this sense exhibits several distinct dimensions. In addition to the straightforward statistical spread across the normal distribution, manifest even in the most homogeneous of populations, we also need to examine the way in which diversity may be structured by powerful underlying variables, such as community and region of origin. As we saw earlier, both the population of South Asia and its Hindu component are far from homogeneous. Hence, there is every reason to expect different trajectories of adaptation for various subgroups: for example, Hindus as opposed to Sikhs; Hindus as opposed to Muslims; Punjabis as opposed to Gujaratis; those of rural origin as opposed to those from urban and professional backgrounds; and quite different trajectories for members of the specific communities that have crystallised in the process of UK settlement.[5] Unfortunately, the census only provides us with some tantalising glimpses of the extent of these diversities. Some of the most relevant are outlined below.

Hindus in comparison with other components of Britain's South Asian population

As Figure 2.3 demonstrates, the Hindu community is far from being the largest component of Britain's South Asian population. Once we combine the Pakistani and the Bangladeshi components – the vast majority of whom are Muslim – with the Indians, as I have done in Figure 2.3(a), Hindus emerge as making up precisely a quarter of this section of the population. If, however, we focus solely on those who identified themselves as Indians in ethnic terms, their salience

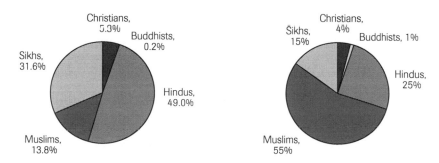

FIGURE 2.3 The religious affiliations of Britain's South Asian (a) and Indian (b) population

becomes much greater: at this level, just under half identify themselves as Hindu, while the remaining half of Britain's 'Indian' population identify themselves as Sikhs, Muslims, Christians and Buddhists (in that order).

Unfortunately the census questions were not designed in such a way as to allow respondents to be further differentiated in terms of their regional origins, which would allow us to differentiate Gujaratis from Punjabis, or those stemming from India's other states and regions. However, the figures do at least allow us to differentiate Britain's Hindus in terms of their countries of birth.

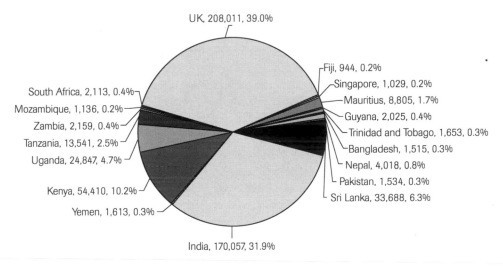

FIGURE 2.4 Countries of birth of Britain's Hindu population

Figure 2.4 shows that the bulk of Britain's Hindu population was born either in the UK or in India; failing that, in other countries within the subcontinent, including Nepal, Sri Lanka, Pakistan and Bangladesh. However, that is by no means the whole picture. The chart also serves to highlight the extent to which the ancestors of Britain's Hindu population had been involved in diasporic activities *before* they moved to settle in Britain. They can be conveniently grouped into three broad categories. Firstly, those who moved west across the Indian Ocean to locations along the east coast of Africa, from the northerly Yemen down to South Africa; secondly, those who moved in an easterly direction to settle in Singapore, Hong Kong and Fiji; and, finally, the descendants of so-called 'coolies', recruited as indentured labourers for sugar estates in Mauritius, Reunion and Britain's most southerly Caribbean colonies.

As Britain's Hindu population has been drawn from a wide range of specific places of overseas origin, it also displays an equally distinctive pattern of settlement in the UK. As Figure 2.5 shows, its members are heavily concentrated in the London area, and slightly less heavily in the Midlands and the South East. By contrast, the Hindu presence in the remainder of the UK is close to negligible.

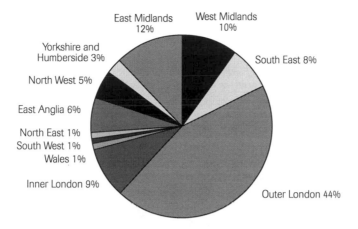

FIGURE 2.5 Regional distribution of the Hindu population in England and Wales

Socioeconomic achievements

In common with most other immigrants, Hindu settlers in Britain had to start at the very bottom of the socioeconomic ladder. No matter what their qualifications or work experience, they had little alternative but to take whatever jobs were available, particularly those shunned by members of the indigenous population. However, Britain's Hindu population is now economically well established. Its older members have spent a lifetime in the British labour market, while their offspring were born, brought up and educated in Britain. This raises the question: 'How are they getting on?'

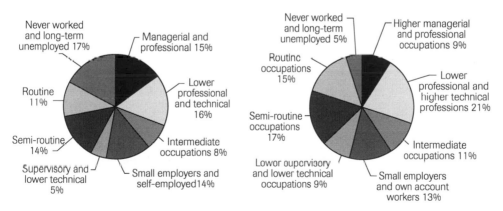

FIGURE 2.6 Occupational distribution of 55–64 year olds in England and Wales in the Hindu population (a) and the population as a whole (b)

If one compares the current occupational distribution of the older generation of settlers – those just about to reach retirement age – with their peers in the population at large, it is evident that the initial setbacks associated with migration have been largely overcome. The Hindu population still contains a substantially larger percentage of people who have either never worked or who are long-term unemployed (and this may be accounted for by the relatively large proportion of women never entering the labour market). Despite this, no less than 15% occupy the top slot in the hierarchy (those in managerial and professional occupations), as opposed to 9% in the population as a whole.

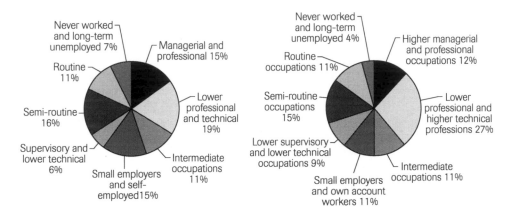

FIGURE 2.7 Occupational distribution of 35–54 year olds in England and Wales in the Hindu population (a) and the population as a whole (b)

Moving on to the next segment in the age spectrum, those described as being in mid-career, we find a similar pattern. This time the numbers in the 'Never worked and/or long-term unemployed' category have shrunk to a level closer to the national average. The proportion of those in the top-most category is still significantly higher than average. On the face of it, those in this age group seem to be growing steadily closer to the pattern of occupational distribution found in the population at large.

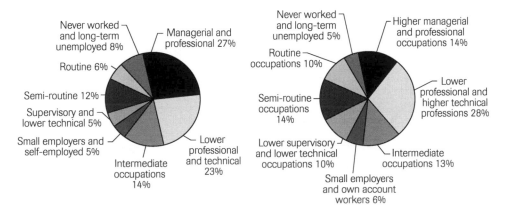

FIGURE 2.8 Occupational distribution of 25–34 year olds in England and Wales in the Hindu population (a) and the population as a whole (b)

However, any suggestion that comprehensive convergence is imminent is immediately refuted when we examine the youngest cohort in the labour market: those aged between 25 and 34. In this age group, the great majority of British Hindus were born and educated in the UK, and are clearly setting off on a trajectory very different from their parents. The leaning towards small-scale self-employment (the corner-shop syndrome), so characteristic of the older generation, appears to be finished. In fact, the proportion of Hindus in this occupational slot has now fallen below the national average. What has emerged instead is a massive increase in the proportion of Hindus found in the top slot of managerial and professional occupations, standing at almost double the level found in the population as a whole.

Conclusion

The message is clear. By dint of enterprise, hard work, and a refusal to 'take no for an answer', Britain's Hindus have overcome the disadvantages and setbacks associated with migration and settlement in an alien land. Members of the middle-aged and older generations have consequently struggled to a position close to, and perhaps slightly ahead of, the norm for British society. However, the socioeconomic achievements of the rising generation of young Hindus are substantially better than that: the vast majority are now moving into professional occupations, and a significant minority taking a further step in their migratory journey, crossing the Atlantic to pursue the wider opportunities in Canada and the United States.

With this in mind, it is worth referring to the achievements of the settlers who established themselves in East Africa a century ago. Despite the inferior position to which they were originally assigned by the colonial elite, by the middle of the century they and their offspring were largely responsible for the prosperity of the East African colonies, within which they then formed the greater part of the commercial and professional elite. But while their material lifestyles rapidly became westernised, their personal, domestic, familial and religious lifestyles remained firmly Hindu. They did not 'assimilate into the mainstream'. In fact, in the context of East Africa's deeply plural society, there was no such mainstream. Instead, they established a multitude of community-specific ethnic colonies of their own. That was the secret of their success. By making the most of the social, cultural, economic and business capital lying at the heart of their own self-constructed communities, the East African Asians pressed their way forward not just on a local level but also globally. In the course of this brief introduction, it has not been possible to explore the *qualitative* characteristics of those resources, but merely to highlight their consequences. However, there is an extensive and rapidly growing literature on the internal characteristics of the multitude of tight-knit Hindu communities, much of which can be accessed through the works listed in the bibliography set out below.

Key points

▪ In 2001, 557,985 British residents identified themselves as Hindus.
▪ The majority of British Hindus trace their origins to India (note that a small but significant number of Hindus are not from Indian backgrounds, but are 'converts').
▪ However, substantial portions of the Hindu population have come not directly from India, but via former British colonies.
▪ Over one third of today's UK Hindu population were born in Britain.
▪ Most Hindus in the UK have roots in Gujarat, with the second-largest group from Punjab. Jackson and Killingley[6] quote the following figures for 1977:
  ● Gujarati 70%
  ● Punjabi 15%
  ● Other 15% (including Tamils, Bengalis, Rajasthanis and Maharashtrians).
▪ The population of Hindus are heterogeneous in terms of their socioeconomic background.
▪ Household structure shows salient features of both an extended family and a larger number of dependent children living with parents.
▪ Within the UK there is a heavy concentration of Hindus around London and slightly fewer within the Midlands (especially Leicester) and the South East.
▪ Socioeconomically, the younger population is taking on more professional and managerial occupations.

References

1 Visram R. *Ayahs, Lascars and Princes: Indians in Britain 1700–1947*. London: Pluto; 1986.
Lahiri S. *Indians in Britain: Anglo-Indian encounters, race and identity 1880–1930*. London: Frank Cass; 2000.
2 Morris HS. *Indians in Uganda: a study of caste and sect in a plural society*. London: Weidenfeld and Nicholson; 1968.
Bhachu P. *Twice Migrants: East African Sikh settlers in Britain*. London: Tavistock Publications; 1985.
3 Mukhta P. *Shards of Memory: woven loves in four generations*. London: Weidenfield and Nicholson; 2002.
4 Ballard R. The South Asian presence in Britain and its transnational connections. In: Singh H and Vertovec S, editors. *Culture and Economy in the Indian Diaspora*. London: Routledge; 2003.
5 Ballard R, editor. *Desh Pardesh: the South Asian presence in Britain*. London: C. Hurst and Co; 1994.
6 Jackson J and Killingley D. *Approaches to Hinduism*. London: John Murray; 1988.

Bibliography

Ballard R. Living with difference: a forgotten art in urgent need of revival? In: Hinnells J, editor. *Religious Reconstruction in the South Asian Diasporas: from one generation to another.* London: Palgrave Macmillan; 2007.

Ballard R. The South Asian presence in Britain and its transnational connections. In: Singh H and Vertovec S, editors. *Culture and Economy in the Indian Diaspora.* London: Routledge; 2003.

Ballard R, editor. *Desh Pardesh: the South Asian presence in Britain.* London: C. Hurst and Co; 1994.

Bhachu P. *Twice Migrants: East African Sikh settlers in Britain.* London: Tavistock Publications; 1985.

Burghart R, editor. *Hinduism in Great Britain: the perpetuation of religion in an alien cultural milieu.* London: Tavistock; 1987.

Centre for Applied South Asian Studies. *Ethnic Plurality and Health* (various papers). Available at: www.arts.manchester.ac.uk/casas/papers/health.html.

Desai R. *Indian Immigrants in Britain.* Oxford: Oxford University Press; 1963.

Firth S. *Dying, Death and Bereavement in a British Hindu Community.* Leuven: Peeters; 1997.

Jackson J and Killingley D. *Approaches to Hinduism.* London: John Murray; 1988.

Lahiri S. *Indians in Britain: Anglo-Indian encounters, race and identity 1880–1930.* London: Frank Cass; 2000.

Morris HS. *Indians in Uganda: a study of caste and sect in a plural society.* London: Weidenfeld and Nicholson; 1968.

Mukhta P. *Shards of Memory: woven loves in four generations.* London: Weidenfield and Nicholson; 2002.

Parekh B, Singh H, Vertovec S, editors. *Culture and Economy in the Indian Diaspora.* London: Routledge; 2002.

Raj D. *Where are you From? Middle class migrants in the modern world.* Berkeley: University of California Press; 2003.

Robinson V. The Indians: onward and upward. In: Peach C, editor. *The Ethnic Minority Populations of Great Britain: ethnicity in the 1991 Census Vol. Two.* London: Central Statistical Office; 1996.

Tambs-Lyche H. *London Patidars: a case study in urban ethnicity.* London: Routledge; 1980.

Visram R. *Ayahs, Lascars and Princes: Indians in Britain 1700–1947.* London: Pluto; 1986.

PART TWO

Issues related to healthcare

CHAPTER 3

The need for cultural sensitivity

Dr Heenakumari Ghanshyambhai Patel, Dr Paul Oliver and Dr Bhanu Ram

Following on from the previous chapters, Dr Oliver and his colleagues broadly examine the practical aspects and implications of Hindu religion and culture in terms of daily life. They explore issues such as language, dress, diet, festivals and alternative care models, with emphasis on their practical relevance to contemporary medical practitioners.

Introduction

For many of its followers, Hinduism is not merely a formal belief system, but a spiritual culture influencing numerous aspects of daily living. These range from basic and well-known lifestyle features, such as dress, cuisine and the mode of greeting to more complex and ethically related matters such as marriage, respect for the environment and approaches to death and bereavement. Within Hinduism, perceived as one of the great 'world religions', lives its rich cultural heritage and enduring traditional values.

This chapter looks behind some of these cultural and worldview issues and examines how they impact on both Hindu patients and their care providers. Hinduism is extremely diverse, and has often been termed 'a family of religions'.[1] It is helpful, therefore, to keep in mind that not all the principles discussed in this chapter will apply equally to all Hindus. However, we hope that a basic understanding of key principles will facilitate care that is more sensitive, understanding and culturally competent. In order to do this, the practitioner needs to become aware of, and subsequently comfortable with, the differences between cultures and, indeed, within them. This will encourage a respectful appreciation of others' beliefs and a more flexible approach to patients of different ethnicity.[2]

A central teaching of Hinduism – and one that significantly influences its predominant worldview – is that the real self is the eternal soul and not the body or mind. In order to provide holistic care, due recognition must be paid to how this influences patient outlook and to meeting his or her multilayered needs: physical, emotional and spiritual.

Language and communication

Hindus originate from the Indian subcontinent, with a landmass comparable to that of the European Union. It should therefore be of little surprise that, among Hindus, regional languages and culture, including communication styles, vary as much as between the English and the French, or between Western and Eastern European. Additionally, many Hindus in Britain are not Indian by birth, but have come via other migrant bases, especially East Africa, thus accumulating even more diversity in communication patterns and health behaviour. Furthermore, not all Hindus are of Indian descent. There is also a relatively small yet significant number of practising Hindus of white or Afro-Caribbean ethnicity.[3–5]

Hindus speak a variety of languages. These include the national language of Hindi, northern languages such as Gujarati, Punjabi and Bengali, and the southern tongues of Tamil, Telegu, Malayalam and so on. A highly significant number, except among the elderly, also speak English. Their fluency in English varies, and depending on the complexity of their health requirements, they may need help from an interpreter.[6] The healthcare provider, and the interpreter, need to be not only sufficiently aware of the patient's cultural and religious background, but also linguistically competent.

Welch[7] recommends that unless the practitioner is entirely proficient in the language of the patient, the interchange should be restricted to a brief encounter. When a family member is the only available interpreter, it is best to focus conversation on the information absolutely needed and to avoid tangential or highly sensitive enquiries. She suggests that the patient's best interest is served by assisting him or her in actively seeking out a healthcare provider who speaks their language. Professional interpreters are to be preferred over family members.[8] In obstetrics or gynaecological care, a female interpreter is preferable, since some Hindu women remain shy about communicating personal issues through a male interpreter.[9]

We would add that even when the practitioner speaks the language of the patient, they also need to empathise with the patient's spiritual and cultural needs.

Naming systems

Another consideration when dealing with Hindu patients is recognising and using specific titles, especially relevant to clients older than oneself as a means of showing respect. Also, particularly when dealing with the opposite sex, titles may also be used out of respect and to protect oneself from any form of sexual indiscretion. The traditional Hindu system is that outside of the marital relationship, each member of the opposite gender is addressed in familial terms, such as denotes a brother (*bhai/bhaiya*), sister (*ben*), aunt (*masi/kaki*), or in a parental mode (as in the use of the term *mataji*, meaning 'respected mother').

TABLE 3.1 Hindu titles

ENGLISH TITLE	HINDU TITLE	USE
Brother	Bhai/Bhaiya	After forename/alone
Sister	Ben/Didi	After forename/alone
Mother	Maa/Mata/Mataji	After forename/alone
Mister/Mr	Shriman/Shri	Before full name
Ms	Shrimati	Before full name
Preacher/minister	Prabhu/Gurudeva/Swamiji	After forename/alone

When completing records, the doctor and other medical staff will need to ensure that certain prefixes and suffixes are not included, as shown in the table below:

Practical pointers: legal names

In Hindu names, out of respect the suffixes bhai or ben, meaning brother or sister, are commonly attached by the patient or family members. Therefore, for example:

Name used: *Suggested format in notes:*
Ramanbhai Patel   Raman Patel
Nituben Shah   Nitu Shah

The husband's first name often becomes the wife's second name and the father's first name is adopted into the child's name.

For example: Mr Jay Patel's wife may be called 'Arti Jay Patel' and the son 'Amit Jay Patel'.

Some familiarity with the naming structure or enquiry from the patient will acknowledge their background and enhance communication. Hindus share the British naming system whereby families share the paternal surname and upon marriage the wife adopts her husband's surname. For men, middle names are often the father's first name.

(Additionally, for a list of common first names, *see* Chapter 4.)

Dress Code: the body as a temple to the Lord

'Don't judge a book by its cover, or a lady by her sari'

Dressed in my traditional sari and ornaments, full of the joys of newly anticipated motherhood, I waited for the consultant obstetrician to arrive for my first antenatal clinic appointment. By my side sat my loving English husband, equally 'expectant'.

The clinic was busy, and as the consultant marched in, his first words to my husband remain with me today, some 24 years on. 'Have you come to translate?' Nonetheless, his obstetrics care was impeccable.

The traditional Hindu dress of *sari* (for most women), and *dhoti* (for men), apart from their unique style and elegance, are spiritually significant, as well as being influenced by historical and socio-political trends. Adherence to dress code varies according to the discretion of the individual practitioner. In Britain (as now in urban India) most men wear Western clothes in public, but wear the traditional clothing when attending a wedding or visiting the temple. This may include the robe (dhoti), as Gandhi wore, or more often a silk *kurta* (loose-fitting shirt) and trousers. Women vary in their preference according to age, background and personal choice, but will usually dress for worship in sari or in the Punjabi *salwar-kameez* (tunic and trousers). However, it is important to note that many Muslim women from Bangladesh wear the sari, and many Sikh women wear the salwar-kameez!

Hindus regard the body as a temple of the Lord and decorate it accordingly. Most people are familiar with the red *bindi* or *kumkum* dot applied to the forehead with vermilion. A married Hindu woman bears the kumkum dot to signify her allegiance to her husband and her meditation for his safekeeping. It is now common for unmarried girls to wear modern decorative versions as fashion accessories, especially when wearing traditional dress. Hindu widows, customarily dressing in white, give up the bindi, but may still apply a *chandan* (sandalwood) paste dot.[10]

Tilak or *tilaka* is a variously shaped mark made on the forehead and, often unseen by others, on the torso and arms. It symbolises the footprint of God, and is believed to safeguard these bodily regions. Tilak is made from ashes, sandalwood or sacred clay from the beds of India's holy rivers.[11] Tilak also helps distinguish the specific tradition of the Hindu patient. Vaishnavas (worshippers of Vishnu) usually sport a mark on the forehead resembling a U, V or Y. Worshippers of Shiva bear three horizontal lines. Many others (including the Shaktas, who worship the Goddess) simply wear a red dot.

There are also certain less well known but important dress items, such as neck beads (*kanthi mala*) and, for men, the sacred thread (*janoi*).[12,13] The neck beads are made from the wood of the sacred tulasi tree, or less often from rudraksha (dried berries). Married Hindu women may also wear a *mangala sutra*, a special necklace of black and golden beads, again indicating devotion to the husband.

The significance is somewhat similar to that of the Western wedding ring, but it is only removed by a widow. Consequently, removal of these items, no matter how inadvertent or well intended, may be considered inauspicious.[14]

On men, the sacred thread, consisting of a number of white or cream strands, is draped over the left shoulder and around the torso. This is also called the *upavita* or sometimes the 'sacred thread'. It signifies initiation into spiritual life and should never be removed without permission, as this may cause offence. During ritual worship, many Hindus tie a red thread on one wrist and continue to wear it for spiritual protection. They may be reluctant to remove it. If removal of such items is necessary – for example, for operative purposes – temporary adjustments can be negotiated, but the patient may wish to seek further guidance from a priest.[15]

These dress items collectively remind the wearer that the body belongs to God. It is also a widespread belief that they secure protection of body, mind and soul. The ancient scripture *Skanda Purana* states that a person decorated with tilak or neck beads need not fear death. Otherwise, without this protection, at the moment of death the agents of Yamaraja (the Lord of death) may come and punish wrongdoers.[16] Sacred items attract divine assistance, such as from the Vishnudutas (the agents of Vishnu) who safely transport the soul to a higher plane of existence. Hence, patients undergoing serious and risky operations may consider these symbolic items highly important.

The Hindu patient may also wear or carry *japa mala* (chanting beads), sometimes in an oval or L-shaped cloth bag. These are akin to rosary beads and are used for mantra meditation, either performed silently or as soft chanting. Naturally, medical staff should respect the rights of the patient to carry and use such items, and their concern to prevent sacred items from coming into contact with places Hindus consider dirty (such as the feet, floor or toilet room).

Cleanliness is next to godliness: the daily routine

Being and feeling externally clean is considered by many Hindus to be important, especially when preparing for or performing daily worship. For example, running water is considered essential for purification, and many elderly Hindus will never have sat naked in a bath full of (what they would consider) their own 'dirty' water. Consequently, shower facilities are more acceptable than the traditional and diminishing Western practice of immersing the whole body in a bathtub.[17] Among the more strict observers, and especially the elderly, a bucket, bathing stool and jug may be the ideal standard. While bathing, mantras or special prayers may be chanted quietly or sung aloud. For many Hindus, other activities of daily living cannot commence until ablutions are complete. Some bathe three times a day before offering prayers at the three junctures of sunrise, noon and sunset. Many Hindus may wish to bathe (or at the very least use a bidet) after passing a stool; otherwise they would consider their subsequent activities to be contaminated. Bathing facilities would ideally be separate from toileting areas. Although not all Hindu patients will be so diligent, medical staff should give careful consideration to cleanliness issues and avoid seeing them simply in terms of religious superstition or 'ritual cleanliness'.

Tearful and upset elderly lady

A 68-year-old Gujarati-speaking woman was admitted with a stroke. She pleaded that her 39-year-old daughter be allowed to stay by her. The request was granted only after a few days of deterioration during which the mother mostly wept, was unable to sleep, felt 'unclean' and was generally found to be difficult by nursing and physiotherapy staff.

She had developed constipation but repeatedly refused to use the commode by her bedside. Previously, she had always had daily ablutions, using running water, and had always been able to wash with water after opening her bowels. Her lifelong routine had been to worship her deities (sacred images) following her ablutions and definitely before addressing any other events of the day. She would not even think of eating before completing her deity worship, which included offering food to her deities. Once her daughter was allowed to stay, she became more relaxed and, as her confidence increased, her mental and physical health began to improve.

Yet, even after discharge from hospital, the idea of the commode in her bedroom pained her. She had her home altar there. She considered it an extra misfortune to have to move her worshipful deities out. The constipation recurred, until some sensitive counselling enabled her to relocate her own bed and commode! By then, she also had a replacement bathing assistant who did not mind arriving early for her ablutions, enabling her to then begin her daily activities.

Vegetarianism: Hindu versions

Vegetarianism was traditionally the norm in many sections of Hindu society, and has been practised for thousands of years. Generations of Hindu families have lived healthily on grains, pulses, vegetables, fruits and milk products. Many first generation Hindus in Britain remain vegetarian; however, there are many, especially in subsequent generations, who are not. Even in theses cases, most still avoid beef at all costs. Hindu scripture reveres the cow as sacred, to be worshipped as one's mother since she provides us with milk.[18] By the same note, the bull, who ploughs the fields and helps provide crops, is respected as the father. In fact, in some traditions the bull symbolises religion, with each of his four legs representing the pillars of virtue: mercy, honesty, austerity and cleanliness. However, the practice of Hindu vegetarianism is significantly different from the conventional understanding accepted in Western culture[19] and it is for this reason that most airlines today provide an 'Asian-vegetarian' option.

Most Hindu vegetarians follow a lacto-vegetarian diet, which includes milk but excludes eggs. In other words, they refuse all meat, fish and eggs, and any products containing their derivatives. They are not usually vegan, so all dairy products, such as milk, cheese, butter and yoghurt, are generally acceptable. Many will also refuse mushrooms and other fungi.[20] Stricter Hindus, especially Vaishnavas, will shun onion and garlic products. Furthermore, some will avoid anything containing alcohol, and caffeine-based products such as tea, coffee and certain soft drinks.[21]

The basis of these dietary choices is the understanding that all foods fall into three categories depending on their qualities. These are the qualities (sometimes called gunas) of goodness (sattva), passion or desire (rajas) and ignorance or darkness (tamas). For example, milk is considered sattvic (of the quality of goodness) and extremely beneficial to healthy development of body, mind and spirit.[22] On the other hand, meat is classified under passion and ignorance and is therefore considered detrimental both to health and spiritual development.[23] The avoidance of meat is also linked with concepts of reincarnation and karma, and the virtue of *ahimsa* (non-violence). It is therefore considered unacceptable to many Hindus, though its consumption is sanctioned in a restricted way by some Hindu texts.[24]

Some medical practitioners may suspect that a vegetarian diet is nutritionally deficient. However, it is important to note that nutritionists in the West have more recently suggested that a vegetarian diet may be helpful in preventing coronary artery disease, cancers and other conditions such as obesity and hyper-cholesterolaemia.[25–31] Medical staff should be aware of their own predisposition towards a particular dietary regime and might respect the fact that a traditional Hindu vegetarian diet, if well-balanced, can offer significant health advantages.

However, if not balanced, Hindu patients may be prone to certain deficiencies such as vitamin B12, calcium and iron. In view of this, and general dietary issues, introductory diet sheets have been provided in Appendix 5, as a guide for clinicians.

Beyond basic vegetarianism, appreciation of a higher consciousness is demonstrated by offering food to God. Such food is known as *prasada*.[32] Thus a select number of Hindus will only accept food that has been prepared at home or at a temple. There is an understanding that the mental and emotional disposition of the cook will affect the nature of the food and, indeed, the well-being of the eater.[33] This explains why some Hindu inpatients insist on their meals being brought in from home.

Food for thought

'Vegetables, grains, fruits, milk, and water are the proper foods for human beings and are prescribed by Lord Krishna (God) Himself.'[34]

'If one offers Me with love and devotion leaf, a flower, fruit or water, I will accept it.'[35]

Problems with compliance

The patient's perception of the content of food or a particular medication may influence compliance. This clearly affects the staff–patient relationship and the patient's response to treatment. There are still anecdotal cases of the elderly Hindu patient getting her 'vegetarian' meal, only to find that it contains egg or fish. This is increasingly rare, but we feel it important to be sensitive to patient needs and recognise that, without diligence in such cultural issues, mistakes can easily be made.

The clinical cases below highlight some of these issues.

CASE 1 Weight loss due to problems with food in hospital

One 70-year-old European Hare Krishna nun was in hospital for four weeks with tropically acquired gastroenteritis. The hospital menu was sensitive, with a vegetarian option, but she confided to us that she lived on a jacket potato with butter, fruit juice, and cereal with milk. Her weight dropped from 65 kg to 48 kg. She observed that the vegetarian soups contained onion and garlic, the cakes and pastry included eggs, yoghurts had gelatine, and many of the salads had dressing with onion and/or garlic, or egg-based mayonnaise. Although she never felt uncomfortable due to the friendliness of the nursing staff, she noticed that when she did not eat anything, they tended to avoid her. She had to rely on her visitors, and those of other Hindu patients, to bring in food from home or the temple.

CASE 2 Iron deficiency anaemia not responding to therapy

Mrs Gandhi, a 38-year-old vegetarian mother of three, was diagnosed to have iron deficiency anaemia. The cause was dietary and she was prescribed iron tablets. Repeat blood tests after two months showed no change in her iron levels or haemoglobin. When questioned, she admitted that she had not taken the iron tablets because they contained a gelatine coating. Advice was sought from the local chemist and the tablet was obtained from an alternative manufacturer. Her compliance and anaemia subsequently improved.

CASE 3 The pharmacists get into the act

A 26-year-old Indian pharmacist, who had previously practised in an Indian, largely vegetarian community in South Africa, revealed that pharmaceutical practice over there allowed her to substitute doctor's prescriptions with equivalent animal-product-free formulations, without needing to consult the prescribing doctors. For example, antibiotic capsules containing gelatine could easily be substituted by suspension formulations of the same drug. However, in her current central London practice, she found it difficult, even impossible, to obtain timely authorisation from the prescriber to meet the needs of vegetarian patients. She commented upon much wastage, as returned capsules could not be reused.

Most Hindus, however, are not fanatical, and will accept essential medicines in warranting situations, and when no vegetarian alternatives exist. This situation may have to be negotiated with the patient or relatives. To increase compliance, we suggest that wherever possible vegetarian alternatives should be sought, especially in day-to-day, non-life-threatening illness. In life-threatening situations, compliance is not usually an insurmountable problem.

> **CASE 4** Gelatine taken by the monk
>
> A *sannyasi* (monk) returned from India with fever and headache. Malaria was promptly diagnosed and the treatment at hand contained gelatine. He was duly informed. The monk explained that his prime responsibility to Lord Krishna and his spiritual preceptor was to take essential measures to care for his body, thus keeping himself in a position to teach, preach and help others in their cultivation of spiritual life. With the non-availability of a vegetarian alternative, he willingly undertook the treatment offered.

Fasting, feasting and festivals

Religious observances, often involving fasting and feasting, are woven into the fabric of Hindu life, closely connected to the religious calendar with its numerous festivals. In these practices, there is a great deal of heterogeneity, underpinned by factors such as individual preference, contextual practicalities, and differences based on regional and denominational background. Nonetheless, there are several widely accepted purposes behind fasting, such as the observance of a vow, the practice of austerity, and the perceived benefits for physical and spiritual health. Fasting also offers opportunity for more focused meditation.[36]

Fasting and feasting are usually performed during festivals (*see* Appendix 2 also) and on other days considered sacred. The types of fast day vary considerably, but can be classified within four broad groups:
1 On the anniversary of the 'appearance' days (birthdays) of Hindu deities.
2 On the anniversary of 'appearance' and 'disappearance' days of important saints (i.e. birthdays and death anniversaries).
3 *Ekadashi/Agyarasa*: bi-monthly observances, on the eleventh day after both the new and full moon.[37]
4 Different days of the week, each of which carries different fasting merits and may be associated with a particular deity.

Fasting varies from a total abstention from all food and drink (including water) to avoiding certain specific foods (such as grains and pulses), or simply eating only once a day.[38] Scriptures advise that breaking a fast routine for health reasons is acceptable, even desirable, and does not constitute a religious transgression. It is well documented that Hindus of South Asian origin are particularly prone to diabetes, hypertension, central obesity and other chronic diseases. Lack of compliance with advised diet and medication may become an issue, especially when patients are fasting or feasting, and appropriate advice should be given at these times.

There is another important issue relevant to festivals. Among many Hindu communities, menstruation is considered a state of physical or ritual impurity, preventing affected women from attendance at the temple, and at certain rites and festivities. Women may therefore come to the doctor, especially during a festival season, to seek clinical help in delaying menstrual bleeding. The uses of either the combined oral contraceptive pill or daily progesterone are generally considered acceptable by both the patient and prescriber for this.

Alternative healthcare models

Today, complementary therapies are relatively commonplace among the general public, and have been adopted by some GPs. Among the Hindu community, use of the ancient Indian system of Ayurveda may be more prevalent. The Sanskrit word *Ayur* means 'long life' and *veda* means 'knowledge' or 'science'. Ayurveda can thus be translated as the 'science of longevity'. It is a system that seeks not only to treat disease but, more positively, provide guidance on healthy living, especially through a balanced diet and regulated lifestyle.[39]

In order to help the patient achieve balance, the Ayurvedic physician is trained in the use of diet, yoga, breath-work, meditation and a vast range of largely herbal remedies. Three main skills are required:
1 determining an individual's unique constitution pattern
2 diagnosing imbalances in that constitution
3 recommending holistic ways to treat those imbalances.

In Ayurveda, a patient's constitution is viewed as a composite of three forces or *doshas* (equivalent to the old Western notion of 'humours'). They are:
1 vata: symbolised by ether and air
2 pitta: symbolised by fire
3 kapha: symbolised by earth and water.

The quality and the relative balance of these doshas determine health and disease. When they act harmoniously, the psychological and physiological functions of digestion, absorption and elimination maintain all-round health. Ayurveda teaches that the body, mind and spirit are intimately linked. Consequently, when a person has, for example, a liver disorder, the physician will focus on far more than that particular organ; he or she will examine the whole body, the patient's state of mind, and dietary and lifestyle patterns.[40]

Many Hindus not only favour Ayurveda but also other complementary medicines such as homeopathy, acupuncture and traditional home remedies. It is difficult to gauge how prevalent the uses of such treatments are, as the patient may not readily reveal his or her use of such therapies. However, explicit enquiry may be needed to fully understand the patient's adoption of such practices.

Doctors and carers need to be aware that professional standards vary considerably in this field.

> **CASE 5** Thyroxine: to take or not to take
>
> A 25-year-old Indian female accountant, born and educated in the UK, was diagnosed with hypothyroidism. Her GP informed her that she would need to take thyroxine over the long term. She came from a family that for generations had consulted a homoeopath. Her father's gout had been 'cured' by the family homoeopath, while the GP had 'only prescribed painkillers' for him. She read lay articles claiming that two patients with hypothyroidism had been cured by homeopathy. She commenced homeopathy treatment and, without informing her GP, discontinued thyroxine. When her symptoms deteriorated, she was reassured by her homoeopath (whom she felt did not approve of allopathic treatment) that 'the symptoms will get worse before improving'. She sensed her GP did not approve of her homeopathic approach. With deteriorating symptoms, she was referred to a hospital outpatient department, where she felt there was more understanding and sympathy towards alternative medical practices. She subsequently felt safest pursuing both treatments simultaneously, hoping that thyroxine would help her in the short term, and homeopathy in the longer term. She admitted feeling very confused at times, as she frequently heard that the different treatments would negate each other. As a consequence, she periodically 'lost faith' in both systems of healthcare.

Key points

- Hinduism is a practical life philosophy, and religious issues cannot be separated from the cultural dimensions.
- Appreciation of cultural issues will facilitate healthcare that is sensitive, understanding and culturally competent.
- The traditional Hindu naming system often causes confusion with medical records. Before adapting the recording of names, to allow easier identification, the legal implications need to be assessed.
- The body is considered to be a temple of the Lord and is therefore decorated with certain items. A patient may be offended if these are removed without consultation.
- Vegetarianism is a widely accepted practice, and acceptable foods do not necessarily coincide with the traditional Western concepts of a vegetarian diet.
- Beyond the basic vegetarian diet, many Hindus prefer that food is sanctified, through offering to the Lord.
- The cow has a special place in the Hindu culture, and practically all Hindus will avoid beef and beef products.
- Festivals, and the practice of feasting and fasting, are an integral part of Hindu

culture, and doctors need to be aware of their impact upon compliance with dietary restrictions and other aspects of healthcare.

ॐ Hindu patients may frequently use complementary therapies, especially those related to the traditional Indian system of Ayurveda.

References

1 Das R. *The Atlas of World Faiths: Hinduism.* Arcturus Publishing Ltd; 2007.

2 Pinderhuges E. *Understanding Race, Ethnicity and Power: the key to efficacy in clinical practice.* New York: The Free Press; 1989.

3 Weller P, Fry E, Wolfe M. *Religions in the UK 2001–03 (Hindus in the UK).* Multi-Faith Centre at the University of Derby in association with the Inter Faith Network for the United Kingdom; 2003. pp. 297–310.

4 Knott K. *Hinduism: a very short introduction.* Oxford: Oxford University Press; 1998. pp. 94, 98–104.

5 Jootun D. Nursing with dignity: Part 7: Hinduism. *Nursing Times.* 2002; **98**(15).

6 Weller *et al.*, op. cit.

7 Welch M, op. cit.

8 Ibid.

9 Jootun D, op. cit.

10 Rosen SJ. *The Hidden Glory of India.* The Bhaktivedanta Book Trust International; 2002. pp. 168–69.

11 Ibid

12 Ibid.

13 Sacidananda Swami, *The Gayatri Book*, Saranagati Edition. Schona, Czech Republic: Vasati Publishers; 2005. p. 101.

14 Shah B. *Mangal-Sutra.* Geocities Online Encyclopaedia internet resource page. Available at: www.geocities.com/Athens/7830/mangalsutra.htm.

15 Sacidananda Swami, op. cit.

16 Bhaktivedanta Swami AC. *The Nectar of Devotion.* Italy: The Bhaktivedanta Book Trust; 1985. pp. 74–5.

17 Knott K, op. cit.

18 Rosen SJ, op. cit., pp. 170–2.

19 Jootun D, op. cit.

20 Weller *et al.*, op. cit.

21 Ibid.

22 Rosen SJ, op. cit., pp. 176.
   Bhaktivedanta Swami AC. *The Bhagavad-Gita As It Is.* Sydney: The Bhaktivedanta Book Trust; 1989. 17.7–10.

23 Bhaktivedanta Swami AC. *The Bhagavad-Gita As It Is*, op. cit.

24 Weller *et al.*, op. cit. Jootun D, op. cit.

25 Segasothy M, Phillips PA. Vegetarian diet: panacea for modern lifestyle diseases. *QMJ.* 2000; **93**(6): 387.

26 Key TJ, Fraser GE, Thorogood M, *et al.* Mortality in vegetarians and non-vegetarians: a collaborative analysis of 8300 deaths among 76,000 men and women in five prospective studies. *Public Health Nutr.* 1998; **1**(1): 33–41.

27 Appleby PN, Thorogood M, Mann JL, Key TJ. The Oxford Vegetarian Study: an overview. *American Journal of Clinical Nutrition.* 1999; **70**(3 Suppl): 525S–531S.

28 Leizmann C. Vegetarian diets: what are the advantages. *Forum Nutrition.* 2005; **57**: 147–56.

29 Sanjoaquin MA, Appleby PN, Thorogood M, Mann JL, Key TJ. Nutrition, lifestyle and colorectal cancer incidence: a prospective investigation of 10,998 vegetarians and non-vegetarians in the United Kingdom. *British Journal of Cancer.* 2004; **90**(1): 118–21.

30 Dos Santos Silva I, Mangtani P, McCormack V, Bhakta D, Sevak L, McMichael AJ. Lifelong vegetarianism and risk of breast cancer: a population based case-control study among South Asian migrant women living in England. *International Journal of Cancer.* 2002; **99**(2): 238–44.

31 Key TJ, Davey GK, Appleby PN. Health benefits of a vegetarian diet. *Proc Nutr Soc.* 1999; **58**(2): 271–5.

32 Bhaktivedanta Swami AC. *The Bhagavad-Gita As It Is,* op. cit., 17.17–10. purport. *The Higher Taste: a guide to gourmet vegetarian cooking and a karma-free diet.* UK: The Bhaktivedanta Book Trust; 2002.

33 *The Higher Taste,* op. cit.

34 Bhaktivedanta Swami AC. *The Bhagavad-Gita As It Is,* op. cit., 9.26.

35 Ibid.

36 Bhaktivedanta Swami AC. *The Nectar of Devotion,* op. cit., p. 64.
Bhaktivedanta Swami AC. *The Bhagavad-Gita As It Is,* op. cit., 6.16.
Krsna Balaram Swami. *Ekadashi: the day of Lord Hari.* Singapore: The Bhaktivedanta Institute Press; 1986.

37 Krsna Balaram Swami. *Ekadashi,* op. cit.

38 Ibid.

39 Rosen SJ, op. cit., pp. 178–9.
Dash B. *Ayurvedic Cures for Common Diseases.* India: Hind Pocket Books Pvt Ltd; 1993. pp. 7–10.

40 Krishnan S. *Understanding Ayurveda.* Available at: www.pioneerthinking.com/insideayurveda.html (accessed 15 September 2007).

CHAPTER 4

Birth and childhood customs

Dr Nilamani Gor

In most religious traditions, birth is considered the start of life. In Hinduism, it marks the start of a new chapter in the soul's ongoing journey through the temporal world. Despite belief that the soul is present in all forms of life, Hindus consider a human birth to be extremely precious, marked by its capacity to promote self-fulfilment and spiritual growth. In this chapter, the author explores and explains the various samskaras (Hindu rites) from before conception to the beginning of adulthood, all aimed to promote the all-round health of the individual – physical, emotional, intellectual and spiritual.

The aim of this chapter is to facilitate better medical care by enhancing the reader's understanding of Hindu birth and childhood ceremonies. Most British Hindus observe rites of passage (samskaras) that are well documented in their ancient holy books, the Vedas and their corollaries. These rites of passage extend from before conception until well after death and this chapter explores those performed up to adulthood.

Samskaras aim to purify the individual and promote an understanding of the purpose of life. They are not simply social observances but help create a favourable mentality for stepping positively from one phase of life into the next, and in moving towards ultimate moksha (liberation from samsara, the perpetual cycle of birth and death). These samskaras, usually 16 in number, are outlined in the domestic section of the Vedas called the Grihya Sutras. Depending on their native location, a family follows one of the various Grihya Sutras. This explains variation in custom between different geographical communities, such as between Gujaratis and Punjabis, or between Southern and Northern Indians.

Mindful of this variety, we attempt to cover in this chapter the primary customs, common to most Hindus.

The ethos behind birth

With belief in the *atman* (the eternal self, or soul) the Hindu tradition reveres all life-forms as sacred. However, a soul taking birth as a human is considered most fortunate, for reasons explained in the Bhagavat Purana:

> One who is sufficiently intelligent should use the human form from the very beginning of life – in other words, from the tender age of childhood – to practise the activities of devotional service, giving up all other engagements. The human body is most rarely achieved, and although temporary like other bodies, is meaningful because in human life one can perform devotional service. Even a slight amount of sincere devotional service can give one complete perfection.[1]

The privileged human birth allows one to enquire about the purpose of life. Such enquiries may lead one on the path of self-realisation, the goal of which is considered *mukti* (liberation) conceived of as a state of 'yoga', or union with God. Upon achieving liberation, the soul is freed from the miseries of birth, death, old age and disease and is reinstated in its original spiritual position: either by merging into the all-pervading brahman (Supreme) or in a personal relationship with the Lord in the spiritual realm. The Vedic literature further states that unless one can train a child for liberation, one should not become a parent.[2] Ideally, it is with this understanding that samskaras are performed throughout a Hindu's life.

Pre-birth ceremonies

The first of the 16 samskaras is called *Garbhadhana Samskara*, literally meaning 'purification of the womb'. This ceremony is firmly underpinned by the Hindu notion of pre-existence, for it occurs before not only birth but before conception itself. It aims to help parents conceive children of sound health, good character and spiritual inclination.

Hindu teachings suggest that unrestricted sensual pleasure causes the eternal self to erroneously identify with the body. For self-realisation, Hindu texts extol the benefits of controlling the mind and regulating all kinds of sense gratification, of which sex is the foremost. Although addiction to sex life is considered a great impediment to spiritual progress, if regulated within the bounds of sanctified marriage, it is considered commendable, as taught by Lord Krishna in the Bhagavad-Gita (7.11): 'I am sex life which is not contrary to religious principles.'

Today, performance of this first samskara is increasingly rare, though medical practitioners are likely to meet couples who practise it to varying degrees.

To begin with, some time after marriage, the couple may prepare for conception and child raising through regular yoga practice, a change in diet and lifestyle according to Ayurvedic principles, and other domestic preparations. The day of conception is selected with reference to the menstrual cycle and to astrological calculations deemed favourable to the child's character formation. On the chosen day, the couple perform worship and sacrificial rites, and chant sacred hymns and mantras to invoke God's blessings for a pious and healthy child.

After this samskara, and subsequent conception, there are two further prenatal ceremonies, which consist of reciting specific prayers and worshipping God to enhance the health and happiness of the mother and child during pregnancy. These are more commonly followed than the former.

The Birth Ceremony (Jatakarma Samskara)

This birth ceremony welcomes the newly born into the world (yet again). A spiritual atmosphere is created by chanting the names of God, such as 'Rama' and 'Krishna', on the understanding that 'the name of God . . . equal to Him, brings all auspiciousness and destroys all suffering'.[3] The subsequent ceremony consists of: purifying the baby with medicated herbs and liquids to assist recovery from the trauma of birth; ceremonial cutting of the umbilical cord; and, recitation of prayers to grant the baby health, intelligence and long life.[4] The father anoints the baby's tongue with jaggery (an unrefined sugar made from sugar cane juice) or honey, often mixed with ghee (clarified butter). According to the traditional Ayurvedic system of medicine, clarified butter is used because it promotes beauty, memory, intellect, talent, lustre, virility and long life. If honey is used (rather than jaggery), Ayurveda recommends purified unheated honey.

However, it is important that maternity staff warn the mother and her partner about the risk of infant botulism.[5] Honey is a known source of bacterial spores that produce *Clostridium botulinum* bacteria. These bacteria, typically harmless to older children and adults, create within an infant's intestinal track a toxin that can cause infant botulism. This condition affects a baby's nervous system and can be fatal. After a baby is one year old, the intestine has matured and the bacteria can't grow. It is therefore advised that honey not be administered to a baby under 12 months of age.

In practice, the ceremony performed in the delivery suite rarely includes all the above-mentioned steps. Most common is the placing of jaggery on the tongue, often accompanied by the chanting of mantras or recitation of prayers in the baby's ear.

The ceremony ends with giving the baby milk at the breast of its mother. Hindu scripture positively recommends breastfeeding up until the age of 12–18 months, or when the mother becomes pregnant again. It is understood that the mother's milk is the best food for the growing infant and designed by nature to suit personal systemic needs.[6] It also clearly helps strengthen the physical and emotional bond between mother and child. Hindu culture emphasises modesty and chastity as essential female qualities, thus implying that women should not publicly expose private body parts, such as the breasts.[7] It is important for health professionals to be sensitive to this by ensuring adequate privacy on wards, as bad experiences may tempt mothers to bottle-feed instead. This may adversely affect milk production, especially in cases of prolonged hospital admission.

To prevent any emotional disturbance caused by envy or other negative, subtle influences on the newborn, it is common for Hindu mothers to apply a small dot of lamp-black *kajol* (mascara) on the child's forehead. Placed just above the centre of the eyebrows, it is intended to divert the attention of strangers from the baby's eyes.

Diet during pregnancy and postpartum

Diet is an important feature of Ayurveda, the ancient system of Indian health-care. Food is categorised in various ways, particularly according to the individual's constitution. Most important is the classification described in the sacred text, the Bhagavad-Gita, in which foods (along with all matter) are classified according to their relationship to the three gunas (qualities, or 'modes'). The three gunas are goodness (sattva), passion (rajas) and ignorance (tamas), which have specific effects on one's physiology, consciousness and behaviour.[8] According to the Bhagavad-Gita (14.8), the purpose of food is to increase the duration of life, purify the mind and aid bodily strength. Such foods are considered under the influence of the quality goodness (*see* Table 4.1). Limited amounts of food in the quality of rajas (such as chillies, or very rich food) are considered acceptable, but foods under the influence of tamas should be totally avoided. Foods under the quality of sattva (goodness) are highly recommended during pregnancy, postpartum and for the weaning child.

Diet is a particularly important consideration after delivery when, according to the Ayurveda, there is an increase in vata (air/gas). The mother should therefore eat foods that decrease vata. Breastfeeding mothers should also avoid vegetables which create gas, as they may cause colic in the baby.[9] They should also eat foods which promote the production of breast milk, such as ghee (clarified butter), barley, wheat, rice, coconut, soups, and spices such as ginger, long pepper, black pepper, cinnamon, cumin, asafoetida, caraway seeds and dill.[10]

Gatrad *et al.* made an accurate observation with regards to foods understood to have hot or cold properties, and breastfeeding mothers use this understanding to help their baby recover from, for example, fever or a cold.[11] Ayurveda explains that aside from this there are also four other factors to consider as they relate to food: (1) qualities, (2) taste, (3) taste after digestion and (4) action on one's individual constitution. Depending on the pathogenesis of a disease, the appropriate substance is used. However, it is not simply a case of using hot foods with colds and cold foods with fever. In fact, during a fever foods with a hot taste after digestion are generally used.[12]

TABLE 4.1 The three gunas and related foods

MODE	QUALITIES	EXAMPLES
Goodness (*sattva*)	Foods that increase the duration of life, purify existence, give strength, health, happiness and satisfaction. They are pure, clean, wholesome, and obtained naturally, without undue difficulty.	Milk products, sugar (in reasonable quantity), rice, wheat, fruit, vegetables, pulses, seeds. Healthy herbs and spices. Meals are balanced, prepared and eaten peacefully with due consideration of health.
Passion (*rajas*)	Foods that give immediate sense pleasure but in the long term cause distress, misery, and disease. They include preparations that are unbalanced: too rich, bitter, sour, salty, hot, dry or burning. They include anything (even *sattvic* food) taken in excess.	Garlic, onion, chillies, pickles, hard cheese, excessive salt and sugar. Meals prepared with hard endeavour, with intention to enjoy, and which excite the senses, tending towards excess and extravagance.
Ignorance (*tamas*)	Foods causing distress, inertia, sluggishness, intoxication and stupefaction; food produced through violence. Meals consist of putrid, decaying and decomposed foodstuffs, including leftovers and anything unclean. Tasteless food also falls in this category.	Meat, fish, eggs, mushrooms, and alcoholic drinks. Irregular meals taken compulsively, to stupefy the consciousness and with no regard for consequences (for self and other living beings). Includes anything eaten in dirty and unhygienic conditions.

Some Hindu mothers will certainly follow traditional herbal and Ayurvedic remedies, and it may be helpful if the medical practitioner is somewhat familiar with them, and aware of their use where applicable. Allopathic practitioners are also increasingly aware of the need to promote health (rather than merely treat disease) through dietary and lifestyle changes; issues increasingly recognised as relevant to children.

The Name Giving Ceremony (Nama Karana Samskara)

To allow mother and baby time to recover,[13] the name-giving ceremony is performed sometime after the tenth day. In the modern world, it is usually performed together with the natal rites (which are technically a separate samskara, in previous times performed on the very day of birth). During the ceremony, the newborn is formally given a name (or names), selected by the parents, the guru or a family elder. The name may be chosen with reference to specific syllables corresponding to the position of the moon in the child's horoscope. Vedic (Indian or Hindu) astrology, called *jyotisha*, is an analytical forecasting system based on astronomical data. It allows the priest to understand behavioural dispositions, and to measure the effects of the past, the influences at the present, and the tendency for events to unfold in the future. During this samskara, the priest or an astrologer may predict the baby's future.[14]

According to jyotisha, the name (or, more technically 'sound vibration') which identifies a person throughout life will have positive or negative effects.

Therefore, by naming a child through astrology, auspicious energies can be promoted.[15] Alternatively, or additionally, it is common for a newborn to be named after a particular deity, saint or holy place, to help them develop godly qualities.

TABLE 4.2 Common Hindu names

Male:	Gopal	Name of Krishna as a cowherd boy
	Vijay	Victorious
	Sunil	'Dark blue' (after Krishna or Shiva)
	Mohan	A name of Krishna, a popular deity
	Anil	Air/wind
	Bimal	Pure
	Jay	Victory
Female:	Arti	Ceremony of lights
	Usha	Dawn
	Punita	Pure
	Sadhana	Devotional practice
	Jyoti	Light
	Nikhita	Earth
	Gita (or Geeta)	Song (often after Bhagavad-Gita)

The First Outing Ceremony (Niskramana Samskara)

This next sacrament prepares the baby for his first contact with the outside world. Traditionally, the baby's first outing is after three lunar moons, thus allowing mother and baby sufficient time to recover after the birth.[16] Although, in the modern context, a baby is taken outside after discharge from hospital, many families still ceremoniously observe the sacrament.

During the ceremony, the baby is first taken to the family shrine and then outside to be in the sun's rays. Prayers are chanted to the environment to request a favourable disposition on the newborn. It is also customary to take the baby to the temple for an audience with the murti (sacred image of God, or of a specific deity), along with an offering of cash, fruit, flowers, vegetables or uncooked grain. Sanctified sandalwood paste called *chandan-tilak* is applied to the baby's forehead, identifying him as a servant of God.[17] The newborn also receives sacred beads, often made of the wood of *tulasi* (or *tulsi*, holy basil), to wear around the neck. For protection, a *kavacha* or talisman may also be tied around the neck with black thread. It is important that the neck beads and kavacha be handled with respect and are not removed or broken, except during emergency treatment.

There have been cases where parents do not wish to bring their sick baby to the doctor before the first outing ceremony, for fear of transgressing their religious duties. However, the Hindu tradition tends to be pragmatic, and health concerns can override rigid practices relating to samskaras, vows, fasting, other dietary issues, and so on. In fact, Hindu religious duties have been classified as: regular (mandatory), desirable (optional) and those performed in a time of emergency. Therefore, health professionals may draw on this understanding to gently persuade parents that children's health should take priority, even from the religious perspective.

The First Grains Ceremony (Anna Prashana Samskara)

This ceremony marks the start of the weaning period and is conducted in the sixth month for males, fifth month for females or at the time when teeth begin to form. The infant is very sensitive during the weaning period. For this reason, during the ceremony, sanctified rice milk pudding is fed to the baby while special prayers are recited.[18] In the weeks prior to this ceremony, specified fruit juices are offered to the child. Since fruit juices are thick liquids, they help in preparing the child for solids.[19] As previously mentioned, foods given to the child hereafter should, as far as possible, be those classified under sattva guna (the quality of goodness).

It is important for health professionals to be aware that teething commonly determines when this ceremony is performed; other indicators include a change in the child's attitude (they may cry in want of food), or an increase in the frequency of milk feeds. This may explain why Gatrad *et al.* found that Hindu babies in Britain are usually weaned at around four months old.[20]

Most South Asian families change from an infant formula to 'doorstep' milk at about five to six months.[21] This is contrary to the Department of Health recommendation, which states that reconstituted infant formulae should be continued beyond six months, to prevent deficiencies of iron vitamins A, C and D.[22] Medical staff should encourage families to adhere to Department of Health recommendations, and there appear to be no religious objections to this.

It is believed that around the time of this ceremony, a child's innate tendencies are beginning to manifest. Hence, during the samskara, a sub-ceremony is often included to ascertain these dispositions. A child is put in front of certain objects, often including holy books, money, food grains and a lump of earth. The infant is then encouraged to move towards the articles to see what they grasp first. Apparently, the baby's preference gives indication as to his or her nature and future vocational tendencies. This ceremony is relatively rare but certainly practised within some Hindu families.

The Hair Shaving Ceremony (Cuda Karana Samskara)

This sacrament is one of the most popular samskaras and involves the first shaving of the child's hair. Almost all Hindu males undergo this rite and, in some communities, females as well. It is considered to remove impurities and bestow keen eyesight, longevity, sound health, strength and beauty.[23] Ideally, the hair should be shaved between the first and second year of birth. In some traditions, male babies are left with a tuft of hair called a *shikha*, situated over the posterior fontanelle of the head. Different reasons are cited for keeping a shikha, most popularly that it gives protection and promotes longevity.[24]

The Piercing of the Ears Ceremony (Karnavedha Samskara)

This rite is performed when the infant is six or seven months old or, alternatively, at the same time as the hair shaving ceremony. While piercing the ears, prayers and mantras are offered to God to grant good health and strength to the baby. Gold earrings are inserted in the ear lobe to strengthen the body and 'give it brilliance'. According to tradition, piercing the ears prevents the occurrence of disease, strengthens the immune system and facilitates bodily decoration.[25]

The Beginning of Education Ceremony (Vidyarambha Samskara)

Performed in the fifth year of life, this ceremony marks the beginning of study, and specifically the alphabet, in preparation for the child's studying of the Vedic (Hindu) holy texts. The ceremony consists of the father or teacher guiding the hand of the child in writing the Sanskrit alphabet. The child is introduced to education along with the worship within the family tradition. Different prayers or mantras may be written during this time for example: the symbol 'om', 'salutions to Ganesh', the Hare Krishna mantra and so on. Again, this ceremony is relatively rare these days.

Religious Initiation Ceremony (Upanayana Samskara)

The word *upa* means 'coming close to' and *nayana* means 'being in the sight of God'. Upanayana is a ceremony which links the child to God through a guru and a lineage of spiritual teachers through which sacred Vedic knowledge is imparted. It was traditionally performed somewhere between the ages of five and 16, but usually around seven or eight years old when the child's personality and character develop. It is not recommended to be performed later since more effort is required then to mould the individual's personality correctly. However, many contemporary families perform this rite shortly before the son's marriage. Some traditions have adopted the ceremony for females, though they don't usually receive the sacred thread.

The ceremony marks the transition from childhood to student life, wherein the boy's natural talent (guna) and occupation (varna) are cultivated. In the ceremony, the child becomes twice born (*dvija*) since the spiritual master is accepted as the father and the Vedas as his mother.

In some cases, the guru is purposefully selected, whereas in others he may routinely be the family priest; in some cases (especially in brahmin families) the father himself adopts that role.

At this ceremony, the child is awarded the sacred thread, which drapes over the left shoulder, and diagonally across the chest. He is also given the *Gayatri mantra*, which he thereafter chants three times a day: at dawn, noon and dusk.

Traditionally, after the ceremony the boy would move away from home to the guru's hermitage for dedicated study. In ancient times, even princes were trained to live simple lives without luxury in order to keep the mind pure and to develop character. The emphasis was on the study of the Vedas, with the aims of becoming an ideal gentleman and citizen. In Britain, this ceremony is mostly widely practised by children from religiously devout families. Medical staff will certainly come across patients who wear the sacred thread, and should be sensitive about requesting its removal (*see* also Chapter 3).

After this samskara, there are three further ceremonies performed before marriage. These are:
1 Commencing study of the Vedas.
2 Shaving the head and/or beard.
3 Graduation.

These three ceremonies are rarely practised these days, though the first is quite often combined with the sacred thread ceremony. Graduation heralds the end of the first of the four ashramas (stages of life) and, for most men, the transition into adulthood and the second ashrama (married life).

Key points

- In Hinduism, newborn children are not 'welcomed into the world' (as in the Abrahamic traditions), but 'welcomed back', and into a particular family and faith tradition.
- The human form of life is considered to be a great privilege, in which one may pursue the path of self and God-realisation.
- To facilitate this process, 16 main samskaras (purificatory rites) are outlined in Hindu scripture. It is important that health professionals have a broad understanding of them and try to accommodate and respect them, thereby improving their working relationship with the family.
- This chapter covers the commonly followed samskara from before conception into early adulthood.
- Diet is a key factor that is traditionally altered during pregnancy, postpartum and at the time of weaning to promote optimum health.
- Doctors should be aware that rigid adherence to some Hindu practices (as surrounding rites of passage) may occasionally be detrimental to the patient's health. They may discuss the options in an informed manner, to be both medically pragmatic and respectful to religious sensitivities.

References

1 Bhaktivedanta Swami AC. *Srimad Bhagavatam.* Los Angeles: Bhaktivedanta Book Trust; 1987. 7.6.1.

2 Ibid., 5.5.18.

3 Sri Caitanya Mahaprabhu. *Sri Siksastakam.* New Delhi: Rasbihari Lal and Sons; 1991. Verse 1.

4 Sharma PV. *Sushruta Samhita.* Delhi: Motilal Banarsidass; 2001.

5 Available at: www.food.gov.uk/foodindustry/Consultations/ completed_consultations/completeduk/acmsfconsult.

6 Harish J. *Dhanwantari.* New Delhi: Rupa and Co; 1992.

7 Bhaktivedanta Swami AC, op. cit., 1.10.16.

8 Bhaktivedanta Swami AC. *Bhagavad-Gita As It Is.* Los Angeles: Bhaktivedanta Book Trust; 1986. 17.8–10.

9 Available at: www.mapi.com/en/newsletters/pregnancy_&_ayurveda.html.

10 Murthy S. *Bhavaprakasa of Bhavamisra,* Varanasi: Chaukhambha Orientalia; 2000.

11 Gatrad AR, Ray M, Sheikh A. Hindu birth customs. *Arch Dis Child.* 2004; **89**: 1094–7.

12 Sharma RK and Bhagwan D. *Caraka Samhita.* Varanasi: Chaukhambha Sanskrit Series Office; 1997.

13 *Sankhayana Grhya Sutra.* Delhi: Motilal Banarsidass; 1987.

14 *Brihat Parasara Hora Sastra.* Delhi: Motilal Banarsidass; 1985.

15 Ibid.

16 *Khadira Grhya Sutra.* Delhi: Motilal Banarsidass; 1913.

17 *Padma Purana.* Delhi: Motilal Banarsidass; 2004.

18 *Gobhla Grihya Sutra.* Delhi: Motilal Banarsidass; 1936.

19 Sharma PV, op. cit.

20 Gatrad *et al.*, op. cit.

21 Aukett A, Wharton B. Nutrition of Asian children. In: Cruickshanks JK, Beevers DG, editors. *Ethnic Factors in Health and Disease,* Oxford: Butterworth-Heinemann; 1989. pp. 241–48.

22 Oppe TE, Arneil GC, Davies DP *et al. Present Day Practice in Infant Feeding: report on health and social subjects.* London: HMSO; 1980. p. 21.

23 *Atharva Veda.* Delhi: Nag Publishers, 1985.

24 Sharma PV, op. cit.

25 Ibid.

CHAPTER 5

Marriage and family life

Dr Vibha Ruparelia

Following on from Chapter 4, Dr Ruparelia explores the journey beyond childhood and starts examining specifically adult issues, related to marriage, family structure, sex, contraception, abortion, infertility and adoption. This chapter draws attention to the understandable tensions between religious ideals and actual practice, between traditional views and contemporary context, and the various ways of coping with these dichotomies.

Introduction

Ethical theories employed in healthcare today tend to apply Western philosophical frameworks to family-life issues, such as contraception, abortion and infertility. However, the diversity of cultural and religious values found in contemporary Britain demand that physicians now be sensitive to the varied perspectives patients bring to professional decision making. Without appropriate social awareness among professionals, cultural differences can result in miscommunication, misunderstanding and less effective healthcare

Many Hindus, particularly of the second and third generations, have become acculturated to Western norms, customs and values. They still bring their own unique perspectives, but are usually quite able to constructively discuss them. However, the issues are more complex, and hence relevant, when dealing with recent immigrants and older people, who often continue to apply more traditional views and values when considering treatment options.[1] However, in both cases, the patient's decisions may be influenced by traditions that share a belief in rebirth, and the concepts of karma and reincarnation, and a holistic view of the person that incorporates the importance of family, culture, environment and spirituality. It is important that medical staff try to be aware of the issues that underpin the views, attitudes and practices of their Hindu clients.

Marriage

A Hindu marriage was traditionally viewed as a union between two families as well as two individuals. Primarily for this reason, Hindu marriages were customarily arranged. The term 'arranged marriage' refers to a marriage that is, at some level and to some degree, arranged by someone other than the couple themselves. The parents – often after consultation with other family elders – initially chose prospective candidates as their future son or daughter-in-law. In most cases, the prospective bride and groom had significant say in the matter. However, there were cases of children being punished or disowned if they did not rigidly comply with parental wishes.

These days, the input from the sons and daughters is much greater. More often, the parents will arrange a meeting with the family of the prospective mate, and the two potential partners will have a short supervised meeting. This leads on to unsupervised meetings and the couple may eventually choose to marry. Very often today, young Hindus make their own selection and subsequently have it approved and blessed by their respective parents.

It is apparent that the hereditary caste system, despite its vilification by many Hindus themselves (*see* also Chapter 1), still operates among many Hindus. Marriages were traditionally not only between members of the same varna (broad social class) but between those of the same occupational subgroup (jati). Marriage between members of different communities has now become far more acceptable, primarily because of increased mobility, urbanisation and educational opportunity. Interracial marriages may, however, often continue to meet with disapproval. It is important to also note that consanguinity in Hinduism is not allowed, as first cousins are also considered brothers and sisters, thus forbidding conjugal and marital relations.

Traditionally for Hindus, marriage was lifelong commitment, allowing only periods of temporary separation (except in the case of *sannyasa*, formal renunciation). Divorce is now no longer unheard of, but remains frowned upon. In most cases where differences have arisen, every effort is made, often with the help of relations and friends, to save the marriage. In situations where a marriage does end in divorce, it will usually be more difficult for the woman to remarry than for the man.

Family structure

Until recently, the extended family structure was the Hindu norm. However, practices in the UK today tend to be far more varied. Traditionally, when a girl was married she would usually join, and live within, her husband's extended family. It is still not unusual to see a household with three or four generations living in the same house. Even when Hindu families no longer live in extended family units, their family responsibilities and commitments often remain relatively strong. Family members tend to consult on many issues. This is reflected where family members contact the medical/social team about the health requirements of another family member.

Most patients are happy for their care to be discussed with certain family members but consent to disclose this information must be sought in advance, as expressed by the General Medical Council.

> Patients have a right to expect that information about them will be held in confidence by their doctors. Confidentiality is central to trust between doctors and patients. Without assurances about confidentiality, patients may be reluctant to give doctors the information they need in order to provide good care. You must treat information about patients as confidential, including after a patient has died.[2]

In these cases, and where possible, the individual's care should be discussed with other family members in the presence of the patient. However, especially within the Hindu community, some relatives may get offended, even angry, if information is not provided, and have difficulty appreciating modern Western norms with regard to confidentiality.

The influence of family elders

Elders in the community are generally highly respected, suggesting to many outsiders a hierarchical structure. Hindu grandfathers continue to act as heads of the family (even from a distance) and elderly women will continue with their domestic responsibilities. In certain situations, however, family pressures cause friction, and a breakdown of the system may cause further tensions within the family.

At present, as extended families diminish, elderly parents often live on their own, in flats, warden-controlled properties and residential nursing homes. This is becoming more common in the UK, especially where work and financial pressure means that no one is at home to look after an elderly parent. In some circumstances, this may also be accompanied by feelings of guilt, exacerbated by social disapproval from within the local Hindu community.

Contraception

With regards to contraception, we see within the Hindu community (as elsewhere) a dichotomy between long-standing traditional teachings and rapidly changing contemporary practices. Hindu texts suggest that sexual intercourse be restricted to married couples and then only for procreation, either by specific intent or consequence. Extra-marital and pre-marital sex is strongly discouraged, if not condemned.[3] With a similar worldview, some Hindus avoid the use of contraception. The main spiritual understanding behind this is that sexual intercourse is specifically for having children to be raised in a God-conscious manner.[4]

Despite these ideals, the norm for most Hindu couples is that all forms of birth control are generally accepted. For this reason, family sizes today tend to be smaller that those in previous generations. However, within the Hindu community, sex is still a relatively taboo subject, or one at least confined to the close family. For this reason, women, especially those who have migrated directly from India, are often too shy or nervous to broach the subject. Therefore, they can be largely unaware of the available contraceptive options.

Contraception: knowing the options

Mrs P came to her GP following a termination of pregnancy. When consulted about contraception she stated she did not realise that there were options other than condoms. She was clearly embarrassed at the time, but since has successfully been on the oral contraceptive pill.

Antenatal screening tests

All pregnant women during their booking visit (their first communication with a midwife or obstetrician) are offered a multitude of tests, including screening for HIV infection and serum screening for Down's syndrome. Hindu culture, and a language barrier, may affect this process. It is imperative that a couple fully appreciates what each test means, and also the implications of a positive result. Where a couple does not fully understand the test and its purposes, they often consider it 'just another blood test'.

It is not uncommon to find a couple unfamiliar with Down's syndrome. In addition, they may erroneously consider the Down's serum screening test to be definitive. Hence it is important that they clearly understand the meaning of low and high risk. Amniocentesis or chorionic villus sampling may be offered, but again the risk and benefits must be clearly stated and understood. Some couples may refuse to have these tests on the grounds that they would not terminate an affected pregnancy. This may, in turn, influence their decision to have Down's serum screening. Maternal age is a risk factor for Down's syndrome. However, recent papers have suggested that the biochemical and ultrasound markers used in screening to assess risk may differ among various ethnic groups.[5] Screen positive rates are lower when ethnicity is not taken into account. In populations where reference ranges for serum screening and nuchal translucency scanning are established in predominantly Caucasian populations, correction for ethnicity is appropriate and can redress differences in screen-positive rates between these different groups.[6]

Part of the screening includes tests for sexually transmitted diseases, including HIV. This procedure needs to be handled sensitively. Sex remains a relatively taboo subject and Hindu women may be too shy to seek help or advice on intimate issues. Furthermore, without both an interpreter and relevant literature (in the right language) the full implications of the tests and corresponding results may be difficult to convey to a non-English speaking couple. If only the negative aspects of a positive result are communicated, a couple may well refuse the test. It would also be unfair to use a child or family member to translate intimate details.[7]

Most Hindus in the UK are of South Asian origin. Estimates at the end of 2002 suggested that people living with HIV-AIDS in South Asia numbered 4.8 million, out of whom 4.58 million were in India. However, although the incidence of HIV is high within India, retrospective studies have shown that HIV and sexually transmitted diseases in this ethnic population remain low in the UK. It is clear that given the steep rise in HIV prevalence across Asia, and the strong links between Asia and the UK, the situation needs to be carefully monitored.[8]

Abortion

Abortion clearly remains a difficult and emotive subject for many women faced with a moral choice in which conscience and religious sensibility play significant roles. Professional circles now recognise that the physician's own religious background can also significantly influence the situation.[9] It is recognised that any medical decision is not taken lightly and can only be legitimately taken with due consideration of the individual's specific situation and their religious leanings.

Among Hindus, there is a wide range of responses. Many accept abortion with little or no reservation; others reject it outright, under all circumstances, on moral and scriptural grounds. Research conducted in Mumbai concluded that 'more than 80% of women disapproved of abortion and 56% thought it a sin'.[10] The scriptures imply that abortion is not permissible and 'count it amongst the most heinous crimes',[11] except where the mother's life is at risk. Purely 'social reasons' divorced from a spiritual or religious perspective (as often seen in the West) seem not to feature in Hindu teaching.[12] That is not to say that Hinduism is not, in some ways, an evolving or world-engaging tradition, nor that it lacks any form of utilitarianism. However, it views life rather differently than most in the West more in terms of its inherent feature of consciousness (and the experiences of the atman, the self) rather than through its external, biological symptoms. Many texts teach that souls enter the womb at the time of conception[13] and that the foetus is a living, conscious being, wanting, requiring and deserving protection. The rights of the soon-to-be-reborn soul have to be balanced against those of the mother and other parties. These points, and the corresponding sensitivities, need to be kept in mind when giving abortion advice to Hindu clients.

The Hindu physician and terminations

One senior obstetrician, when asked about her reasons for refusing to take part in terminations, explained: 'The foetus is considered a vulnerable and dependent living entity in need of protection. The scriptures further elaborate that where a termination of pregnancy is carried out, not only does that soul suffer by needing to seek another womb, but also the mother and physician suffer by being involved in the termination.'

One specific problem, prevalent within parts of India, is prenatal sex selection for non-medical reasons; that is, choosing termination based on the gender of the foetus.[14] Some claim that the preference Hindus have for sons is based on religious reasons, such as the need to have a male offspring to offer the rites after death;[15] others dispute this, claiming that the problem is purely socioeconomic, often based on consideration of paying a substantial dowry when daughters get married. However, according to most Hindus, the overriding religious perspective is based on the perception of the soul and the corresponding notion of ahimsa (non-violence). There is also a case for suggesting that such prenatal sex selection is only morally repugnant if abortion itself is wrong – as indeed many Hindus themselves believe. Although prenatal sex selection is relatively rare within the UK (as compared to India), it may occur and clinicians need to be aware of this and take appropriate steps, such as refusing to reveal the sex of the baby.

Looking now at the practical issues, prenatal diagnosis involves an early invasive procedure, such as chorionic villus sampling, between 10 and 14 weeks of gestation or, in the later stages, ultrasonography or amniocentesis. The earliest that foetal sex can be determined reliably by ultrasound is 16 weeks. Conventionally in the UK, ultrasounds are performed for dating the pregnancy at 12–15 weeks and then a second is performed at about 20 weeks to check for foetal anomalies. Therefore, the dating scan is not particularly reliable in determining foetal sex and the later anomaly scan would provide the information very late in the pregnancy. Legally, abortions can be performed up until 24 weeks of gestation, but, after 12 weeks, and particularly after 15 weeks, a medical, as opposed to a surgical, termination of pregnancy would be recommended in the UK.[16] Most hospitals in the UK do not disclose the sex of the foetus at scanning. To bypass this impediment, some Asian couples seem to be returning to India to have a pregnancy aborted if the foetus is confirmed to be female.[17]

The issue has also been recognised by the Human Fertilisation and Embryology Authority, which has reaffirmed its position of opposing sex selection for such non-medical reasons.[18] In India, proposals are being put forward to register all pregnant women with the government and for them to seek permission to undergo an abortion. This is to stop abortion of an unwanted female foetus.[19]

Trying for a boy?

Ritu says two of her aunts in Britain have had five abortions between them in their quest for a boy. Both were eventually refused ultrasound tests in Leicester and had them privately.

'There are clinics in Leicester that won't identify the sex of babies to Asian women. They have a policy, they say, so more British Asians are coming to India when they are pregnant to make sure everything goes to plan. All I want to do is keep my family happy. My husband doesn't seem to care. We already have two daughters and he agrees with his mother that we need a boy, so I'm going through with it; I don't have any choice. We are going on holiday after this and we will try again for a boy.'[20]

Infertility

'Often the sexual act fails to produce pregnancy at all. So although all parents desire a beautiful, highly qualified child, this is often not the case. Thus it can be understood that ultimately it is by the mercy of the Supreme Lord that a man and woman are able to produce a child by the sexual act.'[21]

Children for most are an essential part of married life and couples are expected to have children. Where this is problematic, it may put strain on the couple's relationship, exacerbated by extended family dynamics and corresponding expectations and demands. The majority of Hindus seem to seek help when having problems conceiving. Some may view it as their destiny, or feel it otherwise inappropriate to seek help. The majority are likely to follow conventional treatments without any religiously based reservation.

For a few patients, decisions may be harder. Some treatments may raise philosophical and ethical dilemmas. Since Hindu texts were written down so long ago, they do not provide explicit and unequivocal guidance on these issues. Couples will probably make decisions largely based on conscience, the application of broad principles, and deliberation over their own particular circumstances.

Treatment that involves sperm or egg donation, or treatment selective foetal reduction, may also be unacceptable on both religious and ethical grounds. Some clients may also disagree with treatment that involves *in vitro* fertilisation (IVF). Currently, after egg fertilisation, two embryos are transferred back to the mother. The remaining embryos are frozen and kept for a further 10 years, during which time the couple may choose to have further treatment. At the end of the 10-year period, any 'unused' embryos are destroyed. Two ethical or philosophical issues may arise here. Firstly, if the soul enters a living entity at the time of conception, what does it experience, if anything, when the embryo is frozen? Secondly, some may consider that destroying the remaining embryos amounts to an unacceptable cessation of a life, akin to multiple terminations of pregnancy.

Although many Hindus will avoid or be unaware of such debates, the medical professional may certainly meet with those who raise such ethical questions. Furthermore, it is important that the process of IVF and embryo storage is clearly discussed with a couple. Sufficient time should be given to them so that they can consider their options and discuss them with a spiritual authority, if they wish, before deciding on the best course of action.

Adoption and fostering

Adoption is acceptable and encouraged within most major religions. Among Hindus, adoption and fostering have long been practised, usually within the extended family and for personal fulfilment, continuation of the family and even spiritual benefit. Total infertility and failure to bear a son are common instances where adoption is practised. By Hindu custom, females become a part of their husband's family, and hence a male child is considered essential to continue the family lineage. In India's history, there are instances where the natural heir to the throne was unqualified and the king would adopt another heir. According to Hindu custom, an adopted male child has the same rights and status as a natural son.[22]

The British Association of Adoption and Fostering (BAAF) has adopted the policy to try their utmost to keep a child in a cultural surrounding similar to, or commensurate with, its heritage, while recognising the unavoidability of exceptional cases. Most Hindu families in the UK will prefer to adopt children from the same cultural and religious background and will almost invariably look abroad to adopt a child.

Going abroad to adopt

Mr and Mrs Patel couldn't have children. They were offered infertility treatment. They spoke to other couples having the treatment and learned about the side effects, time and expense involved. They were quoted a 23% chance of having a baby with IVF.

They looked into adoption. The UK waiting list for an Asian child was up to 11 years and they had no guarantee that the child would not be of mixed race. They wanted the baby to be Gujarati as they were, though they weren't concerned about the child's caste.

They went to an orphanage near the place Mrs Patel was from in Gujarat and brought a baby girl to England for adoption. Baby Amy had been given up for adoption by her parents as she was their third daughter and they couldn't afford her dowry. Mr and Mrs Patel had applied to social services to adopt a baby from India and the whole process took about three years.

They were overjoyed when they gained custody. Mrs P says, 'God gave me a gift.'

The child with disability or special needs

The Hindu law books called *Dharma-Shastra* clearly support deferential treatment of the sick and disabled in a number of important social and legal contexts; for example, they are exempt from taxation and enjoy a degree of legal immunity. The ideal is that the elderly and the mentally or physically disabled are never excluded from the family but are sheltered within it. Indeed, among the Hindu community, families who abandon those in need may meet with social disapproval. Caring for a disabled person is considered an act of charity. Nevertheless, Hindu families, like all others, will face the same emotional and lifestyle changes when looking after a disabled relative.

Stillbirth and neonatal death

Another instance requiring professional cultural sensitivity is with regard to neonatal death and stillbirth. Although cremation is the Hindu norm – prompting any lingering soul to move on to its next body – exception is made in the case of those considered sinless; saints, babies (including the stillborn) and children under around the age of five (though different traditions will disagree on the precise age). Their bodies are usually buried rather than cremated.[23] With the stillborn, some families may prefer to bathe and prepare the baby's body themselves, often sprinkling it with water from sacred rivers such as the Ganga (River Ganges) and decorating the baby's body with chandan (sandalwood paste and clay from sacred rivers). It is important that medical staff are sensitive to the family's wishes to perform such ceremonies.

Key points

- Hindu marriages are seen as a union between two families and to some degree may still be arranged or assisted.
- Although extended family structures have not always remained the social norm, within Britain family ties still tend to be relatively strong.
- Within the Hindu community (as elsewhere) there are tensions between traditional teachings and contemporary practice, particularly with regard to contraception and abortion, and there may be issues to do with resultant feelings of guilt.
- Hindus tend to look abroad for adoption, as they often prefer to adopt children from similar cultural and religious backgrounds.
- Most infertility treatments are acceptable to the majority of Hindus.
- Adoption and fostering are acceptable and encouraged.
- Stillborn and neonate corpses are buried rather than cremated.
- With stillborn children, doctors should be aware that parents may wish to perform some ceremony for the soul of the baby.

References

1 Coward H and Sidhu T. Bioethics for clinicians: 19. Hinduism and Sikhism. *CMAJ.* 2000; **163**(9): 1167–70.

2 *Confidentiality: protecting and providing information.* UK: General Medical Council; 2004.

3 Menski W. Hinduism. In: Morgan P, Lawson C, editors. *Ethical Issues in Six Religious Traditions.* Edinburgh: Edinburgh University Press; 1996. p. 20.

4 Bhaktivedanta Swami AC. *The Bhagavad-Gita As It Is.* Los Angeles: The Bhaktivedanta Book Trust; 1986. p. 741.

5 Spencer K, Heath V, El-Sheikhah A, *et al.* Ethnicity and the need for correction of biochemical and ultrasound markers of chromosomal anomalies in the first trimester: a study of Oriental, Asian and Afro-Caribbean populations. *Prenatal Diagnosis.* 2005; **25**(5): 365–9.

O'Brien JE, Dvorin E, Drugan A, *et al.* Race-ethnicity-specific variation in multiple-marker biochemical screening: alpha-fetoprotein, hCG, and estriol. *Obstet Gynecol.* 1997; **89**(3): 355–8.

6 Ibid.

7 Lewis G, editor. *Why Mothers Die 2000–2002: report on confidential enquiries into maternal deaths in the United Kingdom.* RCOG Press; 2004. Chapter 18.

8 Health Protection Agency. *Mapping the Issues: HIV and other sexually transmitted infections in the United Kingdom.* HPA; 2005.

Sethi G, Lacey CJ, Fenton KA, *et al.* South Asians with HIV in London: is it time to rethink sexual health service delivery to meet the needs of heterosexual ethnic minorities? *Sex Transm Infect.* 2004; 80: 75–7.

Cliffe S, Mortimer J, McGarrigle C, *et al.* Surveillance for the impact in the UK of HIV epidemics in South Asia. *Ethnicity and Health.* 1999; **4**(1–2): 5–18.

9 University of Chicago. Conscience, religion alter how doctors tell patients about options. *ScienceDaily.* 8 February 2007. Available at: http://www.sciencedaily.com/releases/2007/02/070208072325.htm (accessed 13 April 2008).

10 Menski W, op. cit., p. 13.

11 Lipner J. On abortion and the moral status of the unborn. In: Coward H, Lipner J and Young K, editors. *Hindu Ethics: purity, abortion and euthanasia.* Delhi: Sri Satguru Publications; 1991. p. 43.

12 Bhaktivedanta Swami AC, *Vedic Evidence, Science of Self Realisation.* Bhaktivedanta Book Trust; 2003.

Menski W, op. cit., p. 32.

13 Das R. *The Heart of Hinduism: a comprehensive guide for teachers and professionals.* Aldenham: ISKCON Educational Services; 2002. p. 38.

14 Sen A. Missing women – revisited: reduction in female mortality has been counterbalanced by sex selective abortions. *BMJ.* 2003; **327**: 1297–8.

Jha P, Kumar R, Vasa P, *et al.* Low male-to-female sex ratio of children born in India: national survey of 1.1 million households. *Lancet.* 2006; **367**: 211–18.

Seth SS. Missing female births in India. *Lancet.* 2006; **367**: 185–6.

Jailing of doctor in Indian sting operation highlights scandal of aborted girl foetuses. *Guardian.* 30 March 2006.

15 Lipner L, op. cit.

16 *The Care of Women Requesting Induced Abortion: Guideline Number 7.* UK: RCOG Press; 2000.

17 Desperate British Asians fly to India to abort baby girls. *The Observer.* January 2006. Fathalla MF. The one hundred million missing females are dead: let it happen never again. *Int J Gynecol Obstet.* 1994; **46**: 101–4.

18 *Sex Selection Options for Regulation.* UK: HFEA; 2003.

19 Zaheer, K. India to register to pregnancies to fight feticide. Available at: http://www.reuters.com/article/lifestyleMolt/idUSDEL1752520070713?pageNumber=2&sp=true (accessed 14 April 2008).

20 Desperate British Asians fly to India to abort baby girls. op. cit.

21 Bhaktivedanta Swami AC, *Srimad Bhagavatam.* Bhaktivedanta Book Trust International. 11.5, verse 41.

22 *Manu Smriti [Laws of Manu].* Delhi: Motilal Banarsidass; 1992.

23 Scott J, Henley A. *Culture, Religion and Childbearing in a Multiracial Society: a handbook for healthcare professionals.* Oxford: Butterworth Heinemann; 1996.

CHAPTER 6

Death and bereavement

Dr Diviash Thakrar and Vipin Aery

In the final chapter, it is appropriate to look at dying and death. To most of us, religion attains importance anecdotally, as when faced with life-altering events such as birth, marriage and death, more so with the last item, and there is already a significant amount of literature that discusses a 'good death'. This chapter aims to enhance the reader's understanding of Hindu approaches to death, with the intent of helping medical and nursing staff offer care sensitive to the specific needs of Hindu patients. These needs extend well beyond the immediate and the physical, and encompass longer-term emotional and spiritual requirements.

Introduction

In this chapter, we explore the subject of death, bereavement and associated customs within Britain's Hindu community, especially as the subject is practically relevant to medical staff. This information is primarily drawn from our day-to-day experience as practising Hindus, as professionals, and as social activists having dialogue with Hindu communities throughout Britain. While our advice is somewhat anecdotal, we believe that our experience offers insiders' authentic perspectives on issues relevant to healthcare providers, and it usefully augments the valuable but insufficient research already conducted in this important field.

Hindu belief regarding death and dying

Hindu theology teaches that the real identity of an individual is spiritual in nature. This nature is described as the real self (or the soul), which is beyond the gross physical body. Birth, youth, old age, disease and death are seen as landmarks for the physical body. The real self, however, does not go through such changes. It neither takes birth nor dies at any time but its existence is eternal.[1]

> One who has taken his birth is sure to die, and after death, one is sure to take birth again.
>
> *Bhagavad-Gita*[2]

Death is thus seen as not only an end to the physical body but also a natural progression of the soul into its next state of existence. The next step may be accepting another physical body, or – as many Hindus aspire to – a state of permanent liberation. This conceptual framework, and the corresponding worldview, may be particularly relevant in the context of counselling; for example, during a terminal illness or in helping the bereaved.

Suicide and active euthanasia

Within Hindu teachings, suicide and active euthanasia are generally prohibited. Broadly speaking, the body is regarded as the temple of the soul, and of God, and is thus considered sacred; premature termination of life represents a violation of the natural law and of sacred trust. Additionally, it is widely believed that it is impossible to circumvent the law of karma, and activities such as suicide not only fail to end suffering but actually exacerbate or prolong it, in this life or a future one. Despite this, Hindu teachings do not encourage undue pain and suffering and where medication is given to improve the quality of life – such as analgesia in a terminal illness – it may be permissible, even with the unintended effect of hastening death. Evidence also suggests that refusing food is sometimes considered acceptable for terminally ill patients.

Final illness

> Whatever state of being one remembers when he quits his body,
> O son of Kunti, that state he will attain without fail.
>
> *Bhagavad-Gita*[3]

Hindu teachings place great importance on the state of mind at death, as a main determinant of the soul's destination, either in taking another body or in achieving final liberation. According to the Bhagavad-Gita, 'One's thoughts during the course of one's life accumulate to influence one's thoughts at the moment of death.'[4] The preparations in the period leading up to death are paramount to Hindus, since they have a significant influence on the mind's state at death. This, in turn, influences the next chapter of life for the soul. For these reasons, many middle-aged and elderly Hindus gradually retire from active life and take their spiritual practices more seriously. During terminal illness, healthcare professionals can help patients achieve solace and avoid unnecessary distress by being aware and accommodating of certain beliefs and customs.

For example, a dying patient may wish to have religious paraphernalia around the bed to help prepare for departure. Common items include sacred images (usually pictures) of deities or saints, sacred flowers and garlands, rosary and prayer beads, Ganges water and religious texts.[5] Most hospitals currently provide a Bible and some a Qur'an, if patients so request; however, a copy of the Bhagavad-Gita (a universal Hindu religious text) is as yet less readily available.

During the final stages of life, many relatives, friends and colleagues may come to offer their respects, comfort the person and give advice on their final sojourn. All parties may take the opportunity to ask for forgiveness for inadvertent offences. In hospitals, therefore, it may be restricting and distressing to adhere rigidly to the rule of only two visitors per bed. Visitors may get offended if they are not allowed to see their dear friends or relatives in the final stages of their life. Priests may also come to give blessings and final instructions to the patient. Chanting of mantras, singing of hymns and recitation of scriptures are common practices to help nurture an appropriately spiritual frame of mind. On the other hand, some patients may require time and privacy for silent prayer and meditation, especially during the early hours of the morning.

Death and dying are clearly a stressful time for the patient and immediate family. During this period, communication and consideration are key issues within the hospital setting. For example, the patient may wish to die at home or, occasionally, leave to pay their final respects at a local temple, and wherever possible these wishes should be respected.[6]

Non-disclosure and final illness

Dying patients may not be told of the closeness of death by medical staff who may find it easier to discuss this issue with relatives and friends, rather than the patient directly. Some members of the extended family may encourage this concealment as they feel they want to protect the patient. The caregivers need to be aware of this and recognise that non-disclosure may lead to possible tensions and residual feeling of guilt.[7] They may want to facilitate a more open discussion and also involve the patient directly. Also, medical staff tend to neglect the spiritual needs of the patient.[8]

Open disclosure and guilt

The Hindu family practitioner warned Ramesh that his father (Suresh) was terminally ill with prostate cancer and tuberculosis. Ramesh did not want his father informed of the prognosis. Unfortunately, the hospital staff repeatedly reassured Ramesh that Suresh would recover, and Suresh was not informed of his impending death. However, as often happens, Suresh was clearly aware that he was dying. Although he gave away his books, talked about dying, and bought a gold chain for his granddaughter's marriage, he colluded with his son's silence. When Suresh died, Ramesh was racked with guilt because he had not been present to say goodbye or to give his father the last rites.[9]

Pre-death rites

Just before a person dies, the family may wish to perform specific rituals. Prevention or tardiness may cause considerable distress to family members, both at that time and for years afterwards.[10] Therefore, it is important to ask family members and close friends how and when they want to be informed of imminent death.

Shortly before death, both the sacred tulasi[11] leaf and Ganges water[12] may be administered to the dying person. Ideally, this is done as near as possible to departure. However, in Britain, this is sometimes performed after death, often at the undertakers and possibly because of impracticalities or restrictions in the hospital itself. This may also reflect the fact that the family members feel uncomfortable or embarrassed in the hospital setting.

Death of a famous Hindu

'Mohandas K Gandhi – his name, Mohandas, means 'servant of Krishna' (God): his favourite book was the Bhagavad-Gita (Song of God): he always kept in his room the Sanskrit inscription 'O Rama' (Oh Lord); and he died with the name of Rama on his lips.'[14]

A dying aunt's last rites

An aunt was dying; everybody knew she was dying. The doctors told the family, and the whole family was present at the death. But when the doctors switched off the life-support machine, they wouldn't let the family give Ganges water or perform the last rites on this woman. The reason the doctors gave was that she would live a little longer, but there was no point, she was dying anyway. They switched off the machine, and they said they must not give her anything that would give her a shock and kill her straight away, that would choke her. But it didn't matter anyway, because she was dying. Even today, 10 years afterwards, it still affects the family that they weren't able to do this. (Gujarati family's story)[15]

In some traditions, great emphasis is also placed, at the point of death, on hearing and reciting God's name, or the name of a particular deity.[13] Visitors may therefore continuously chant or sing prayers and mantras (such as the names of Rama, Krishna, or the sacred syllable 'om'). Unless there are clear counterindications, relatives and other attendees should be permitted to help create, in a manner respectful to others in the vicinity, an auspicious atmosphere for the departing soul.

Death rites (Antyeshti Samskara)

Following death, it is customary that immediate family members close the mouth and eyes of the deceased, and straighten the arms. After transferring the corpse to the undertakers, they wash and dress it (sometimes in traditional dress). To avoid the associated distress, relatives these days often ask the undertakers to perform these duties. From here on, preparations are made for the cremation. On the day itself, the body is usually returned to the home of the deceased for a few hours, allowing the priest to perform the final ceremony, and friends and relatives to offer respects. The body is then taken to the cremation ceremony, in which final prayers and tributes are offered.

Cremation is considered important as it apparently breaks the attachment between the soul and its recently relinquished body. Burning is also considered a purifying process. Burials are acceptable and commonplace practice for children under the age of 27 months[16] (or, in some traditions, under five years old) and for saints and other exceptionally pious or holy people.[17] After cremation, a relative such as the eldest son collects the ashes and takes them for dispersion in sacred rivers such as the Ganges or Yamuna, while a priest leads a final ceremony. It is widely believed that contact of the ashes with sacred water ensures liberation for the departed soul. Nowadays in Britain, many second and third generation Hindus use local rivers, such as the Thames and Severn.

In India, the time span from death to cremation is usually only a matter of hours. Ideally, a death during the day warrants a cremation before dusk, and a night departure requires a cremation before dawn. In Britain, this process takes at best three to four days. Measures to ensure that it is not unnecessarily prolonged may greatly reduce any concomitant distress for the family.

Period of mourning

Following death, there is a specified period of purification and mourning. This period generally lasts for 13 days, though there is some variation according to region, tradition and family background. This is a period for social support, family bonding and expression of grief. Each evening, family members and friends gather for prayers and meditation on behalf of the deceased. During this time, family members may also refrain from certain foodstuffs, such as sweets. They may also be restricted from entering the temple or performing rituals, as they are considered temporarily impure. On the thirteenth day, a ceremony ends the official period of contamination and purification.[18] Carers should note that after this date the bereaved is more prone to isolation, often making bereavement reactions more pronounced.

However, the relationship between the deceased and family does not end here. Within the annual Hindu calendar there is a 15-day period called shraddha, during which the forefathers are honoured.[19] The aim of these observances, which include acts of charity and ceremonies led by a priest, is primarily to help the departed soul in its spiritual progress.

The process of grieving

'The individual soul is unbreakable and insoluble, and can be neither burned nor dried. He is everlasting; present everywhere, unchangeable, immovable and eternally the same.'[20]

'It is said that the soul is invisible, inconceivable and immutable. Knowing this, you should not grieve for the body.'[21]

'Thereafter the Pandava princes, desiring to offer water to the dead relatives, went to the Ganges. . . . Having lamented over them and sufficiently offered Ganges water, they bathed in the Ganges, whose water is sacred due to being mixed with the dust of the lotus feet of Lord Krishna.'[22]

Framework for understanding bereavement

There is limited biomedical literature on the grieving process within Hinduism, and some professional concern that current models of bereavement management are not entirely relevant to the Hindu patient.[23] There is even a call to have a more structured approach to care of bereaved patients in the primary care setting.[24] Present provisions in general practice appear to be patchy and inconsistent, and broad evaluative research suggests that most studies inordinately concentrate on the attitudes of the GP and are thus insufficiently focused on the wishes of the patient.[25] Clearly, more research is needed on how the patient's cultural and religious beliefs affect the grieving process.

Post-mortems

Although most Hindus make no formal objection to post-mortems, it can still be very distressing for the family.[26] It is helpful if mortuary staff understand the experiences and cultural perspectives of Hindu families. Mortuary staff working with South Asian patients have noted the stitching and presentation of the body after the post-mortem is very variable, depending more on which hospital the body comes from rather than the cause of the autopsy. Considering that the body is usually washed and clothed by family members, poor presentation of the body can be very distressing. Care is therefore needed with the presentation of the body after a post-mortem.

Poor presentation

Even a doctor who went to the mortuary to see his father's body after the post-mortem was shaken to find that the incision, which had been crudely stitched up, had not been covered.[27]

Organ transplant

Today, the demand for transplant organs far outstrips the supply, a phenomenon which research reveals to be more pronounced among the South Asian population.[28] Some commentators have suggested that religious traditions have prevented South Asians from donating organs; however, there appear to be no clear objections by most Hindus.[29] Hindu teachings, with their ancient foundations, make no direct reference to contemporary organ transplants. Hence, moral concerns are more or less a matter for the individuals concerned. Those involved in the organ requests process should be aware that the religion does not seem to explicitly deter the patient from donating.[30] Healthcare professions requesting donations from the Hindu community need not be reluctant to ask, although it is possible that some adherents may have personal reservations.

Key points

- Hindus believe that the individual's true identity is as an eternal soul (the atman, or 'real self'). Death is thus seen as a transition from one state of existence to the next.
- The ultimate aim of a 'good death' is to escape the cycle of birth and death and to return to God.
- There are important spiritual practices and rites of passage (samskaras) to be performed before and after death. If these are prohibited, it can cause considerable distress to both the dying patient and the family.
- Hinduism forbids both suicide and active euthanasia.
- There is limited biomedical literature on the grieving process within Hinduism, although there is a traditional belief that the release of grief and pent-up emotions are necessary for sound health.
- Current models of bereavement may not be relevant to the Hindu patient.
- After death, the body is cremated, except in certain cases, as with saints and infants.
- Care is needed in the presentation of the body after post-mortem.
- Organ donation and transplantation are not explicitly prohibited within Hinduism.

References

1 Bhaktivedanta Swami AC. *Bhagavad-Gita As It Is*. Los Angeles: Bhaktivedanta Book Trust; 1989. 2.20.

2 Ibid., 2.27.

3 Ibid., 8.6.

4 Ibid., 8.6 purport.

5 Wood E, Subrahmanyam SV. *The Garuda Purana (Saroddhara)*. Berkeley: University of California Press; 1988. 9.31.

6 Bhaktivedanta Swami AC. *Srimad Bhagavatam*. Los Angeles: Bhaktivedanta Book Trust; 1987. 11.18.5. purport.

7 Firth S. End-of-life: a Hindu view. *Lancet*. 2005; **682**: 86.

8 Kmietowicz Z. Nearly half of all patients dying in English hospitals are not aware they have only hours to live. *BMJ*. 2007; **335**: 1176.

9 Firth, End-of-life, op. cit.

10 Firth S. *Dying, Death and Bereavement in the British Hindu Community*. Bondgenotenlaan, Leuven: Utigeverji Peeters; 1997. p. 69.

11 Wood E, Subrahmanyam SV, op. cit., 9.9.

12 Ibid., 9.22.

13 Ibid., 8.9.

14 Prime P. *Hinduism and Ecology*. Delhi: Motilal Banarsidass; 1994. p. 60.

15 Firth S. *Dying, Death and Bereavement in the British Hindu Community*. op. cit., p. 117.

16 Wood E, Subrahmanyam SV, op. cit., 10.93.

17 Ibid., 10.102.

18 Ibid., 13.28.

19 Ibid., 13.106.

20 Bhaktivedanta Swami AC, *Bhagavad-Gita As It Is*, op. cit., 2.24.

21 Ibid., 2.23–25.

22 Bhaktivedanta Swami AC, *Srimad Bhagavatam*, op. cit., 1.8.1–2.

23 Woof WR, Carter YH. The grieving adult and the general practitioner: a literature review in two parts (part 1). *British Journal of General Practice*. 1997; **47**: 443–8. Woof WR, Carter YH. The grieving adult and the general practitioner: a literature review in two parts (part 2). *British Journal of General Practice*. 1997; **47**: 509–14.

24 Charlton R, Dolman E. Bereavement: a protocol to primary care. *British Journal of General Practice*. 1995; **45**: 427–30.

25 Main J. Improving management of bereavement in general practice based on survey of recently bereaved subjects in a single general practice. *British Journal of General Practice*. 2000; **50**: 863–7.

26 Firth, *Dying, Death and Bereavement in the British Hindu Community*, op. cit., p. 129.

27 Ibid., p. 130.

28 Trivedi HL. Hindu religious views in context of transplantation of organs from cadavers. *Transplant Proc*. 1990; **22**: 942.

29 Randhawa G. The impending kidney transplant crisis for the Asian population in the UK. *Public Health*. 1998; **112**: 265–8.

30 Randhawa G. Enhancing the health professional's role in requesting transplant organs. *British Journal of Nursing*. 1997; **6**(8): 429–34. Randhawa G. Exploratory study examining the influence of religion on organ donation amongst the Asian population in Luton, UK. *Nephrology Dialysis Transplantation*. 1998; **13**: 1949–54.

Important Hindu deities

Rasamandala Das

There are three main deities, who are collectively called 'the Trimurti'. They are Brahma (the creator), Vishnu (the preserver) and Shiva (the destroyer). Each has a wife, and these are the three main goddesses. From these six, we can also identify the three main focuses of worship, which correspond to the three great Hindu communities (Vaishnavas, who worship Vishnu; Shaivas, who worship Shiva; and Shaktas, who worship Shakti).[1] This list can be extended by adding another six popular deities, making a total of 12. A further six who were commonly worshipped in ancient times have been added at the bottom.

Trimurti
- **Brahma** – the Creator.
- **Vishnu** – the Preserver.
- **Shiva** – the Destroyer.

Wives of the Trimurti
- **Sarasvati** – Goddess of Learning, wife of Brahma.
- **Lakshmi** – Goddess of Fortune, wife of Vishnu.
- **Shakti** – Mother Nature, wife of Shiva.[2]

Related to the Trimurti
- **Rama** – form or avatar of Vishnu; his wife is Sita.
- **Krishna** – form or avatar of Vishnu; consort is Radha.

- **Hanuman** – servant of Rama and Sita.
- **Ganesh** – remover of obstacles; son of Shiva and Shakti.
- **Skanda** – god of war; son of Shiva and Shakti.[3]
- **Surya** – sun god; a form of Narayan (Vishnu).

Other deities with roles in universal management

- **Indra**– rain-god and king of heaven.
- **Chandra** – moon god.
- **Agni** – god of fire.
- **Vayu** – wind god.
- **Varuna** – god of the waters.
- **Yama** – god of death and justice.[4]

Notes

1 Brahma, though one of the Trimurti, is rarely worshipped.
2 Parvati, Durga and Kali are all forms of Shakti.
3 Skanda is also known as Murugan, Karttikeya and Subramaniam.
4 Not all Hindu groups have the same opinions about the above deities and their respective positions. For example, members of ISKCON consider Krishna to be the source of Vishnu and his avatars (rather than vice versa); the largest Swaminarayan group, the BAPS Swaminarayan Sanstha, considers Bhagavan Swaminarayan to be the source of Vishnu; and some Hindus believe the Supreme to be a formless, impersonal force and that all deities are equal, or even imaginary.

Twelve important festivals

Rasamandala Das

NAME OF FESTIVAL	DATES	DETAILS
1 Sarasvati Puja	19/1–17/2	Worship of Sarasvati, the goddess of learning; it coincides with Vasant-panchami, which marks the start of spring; Hindu celebrants dress in yellow cloth.
2 Maha Shiva Ratri	12/2–12/3	Important festival for the worshippers of Shiva. In India, festivities often continue throughout the night. The image of Shiva is offered milk and bilva leaves.
3 Holi	28/2–28/3	Hindus douse each other with coloured water and powders; also connected to the half-man/half-lion incarnation of Vishnu. Bonfires are lit to commemorate the story.
4 Rama Navami	24/3–23/4	Birthday of Rama, one of the two principal avatars (incarnations) of Vishnu, whose exploits are retold in the Ramayana. His wife, kidnapped by Ravana, is called Sita.
5 Hanuman Jayanti	29/3–28/4	Birthday of Hanuman, the monkey warrior and devoted servant of Rama and Sita. He is also worshipped in his own right, especially by soldiers and sportsmen.
6 Raksha Bandhana	1/8–30/8	A family festival in which girls tie lucky amulets on the wrists of brothers (and other male relatives), who promise to protect their sisters in return.
7 Janmashtami	12/8–10/9	A festival in honour of the birth of Lord Krishna, one of the most popular of all deities. Hindus fast until midnight, the time of Krishna's birth, when there is a gorgeous arti (greeting) ceremony.

continued.

NAME OF FESTIVAL	DATES	DETAILS
8 Ganesh Chaturthi	24/8–22/9	A widely popular festival celebrating the birth of Ganesh, one of Shiva and Parvati's two sons. Huge images are paraded through the streets and finally immersed in water.
9 Navaratri	18/9–17/10	The festival of nine nights. During the day ritual fire ceremonies are performed. Hindus gather each evening to honour Shakti (Shiva's wife) and other goddesses, and to perform the famous circle and stick dances.
10 Durga Puja	24/9–23/10	Durga is a warlike and protective aspect form of Shakti, especially popular in Bengal, Punjab and Jammu Kashmir. She is worshipped in a form with 10 arms, carrying an assortment of weapons and riding upon a lion.
11 Dussehra	27/9–26/10	Festival celebrating Rama's victory over the evil 10-headed king called Ravana. It involves burning huge effigies of this anti-hero.
12 Diwali	17/10–15/11	Diwali is celebrated by decorating houses and temples with rows of divas (lamps). It is associated with Rama, and with Lakshmi, goddess of wealth, who is worshipped at this time. The day after Diwali marks the new year for many Hindus.

Notes

1 The dates vary each year according to the Gregorian calendar, and shown here are the earliest and latest possible dates. In the case of festivals spanning several days, these dates usually refer to the first day.

2 Some communities have their own predominant, more exclusive festivals. For example, for the BAPS Swaminarayan Sanstha, this is the appearance day of Bhagavan Swaminarayan; for ISKCON, the appearance day of Chaitanya; and for the Ramakrishna Mission, the birthdays of Ramakrishna and Vivekananda.

Important Hindu groups represented in the UK

Rasamandala Das

The Swaminarayan Tradition

Sahajanand Swami (1781–1830), later known as Swaminarayan, founded the Swaminarayan tradition of Hinduism in the early 19th century. Devotees, who are largely from Gujarat, worship Swaminarayan as God and follow a Vaishnava form of devotion. There are various Swaminarayan groups with different views on the identity of the guru and the authentic line of succession. The largest is BAPS Swaminarayan Sanstha, whose current leader is Pramukh Swami and which is well known for its elaborate traditional temple in Neasden, London.

The Hare Krishna Movement (ISKCON)

The International Society for Krishna Consciousness is a strand of Bengali Vaishnavism following the devotional saint Chaitanya (1486–1534). He taught devotion to a personal God (Krishna) through the congregational chanting of the Hare Krishna Mantra. ISKCON was founded in 1966 by Bhaktivedanta Swami. The movement, now well established throughout the world, is well known for its sari-clad and saffron-clothed Western followers.

Ramakrishna Mission

The Ramakrishna Mission was founded by the Bengali Vivekananda Swami (1863–1902) in the name of his guru, Ramakrishna (1836–86). It teaches the *advaita* version of Vedanta philosophy coming from Shankara. It is headed by a well-disciplined and organised body of sannyasis. It is still particularly popular in Bengal and has centres worldwide.

Pushti Marg

The Pushti Marg (path of nourishment) tradition originated with the bhakti (devotional) revivalist Vallabha (1479–1531). Its followers place much emphasis on home worship, especially of Krishna in his form as an infant. Many of its members are from the Lohana business community, hailing from Gujarat.

The Arya Samaj

Members of the Arya Samaj follow the teachings of the reformer Dayananda Sarasvati (1824–83), who rejected the practices of caste and murti worship. Their main ceremony is the *havan* (sacred fire ceremony). They remain influential worldwide, and in Britain, where most followers come from the Punjabi community.

Other leaders and groups

There are a number of other influential Hindu leaders, including Sri Ravishankar, founder of the highly popular 'Art of Living' movement, and Amritanandamayi, affectionately called 'Amma' and known as India's 'hugging saint'. There are also several organisations which do not strictly classify themselves as Hindu but which are clearly related. These include:

- The Satya Sai Baba Organisation, headed by Sai Baba, considered a reincarnation of the saint Kabir. The organisation understands itself as a spiritual organisation which embraces all faiths. It has centres throughout the UK.
- Transcendental Meditation, which rocketed to popularity in the 1960s under the leadership of Maharishi Mahesh Yogi. It teaches mantra meditation and remains popular today.
- The Brahma Kumari Worldwide University, founded in 1931 by Brahma Baba, and well known for its work with the United Nations. Its members are predominantly women.

Umbrella organisations

Important umbrella organisations include the National Council for Hindu Temples, the Hindu Council UK and the Hindu Forum of Britain.

(Contact details based on websites as of 2 January 2008.)

National Council of Hindu Temples
The Secretary
The National Council of Hindu Temples (UK)
Shree Sanatan Mandir
84 Weymouth Street
off Catherine Street
Leicester
LE4 6FQ
Tel: 0116 266 1402
E-mail: info@nchtuk.org
www.nchtuk.org/

Hindu Council UK
Boardman House
64 Broadway
Stratford
London E15 1NT
Tel: 020 8432 0400
E-mail: admin@hinducounciluk.org
www.hinducounciluk.org/newsite/index.asp

Hindu Forum of Britain
Unit 3, Vascroft Estate
861 Coronation Road
Park Royal NW10 7PT
Tel: 020 8965 0671
E-mail: info@hfb.org.uk
www.hfb.org.uk/

Educational centres

(Contact details based on websites as of 2 January 2008.)

Institute for Indian Art and Culture – Bharatiya Vidya Bhavan
4a Castletown Road
West Kensington
London W14 9HE
Tel: 020 7381 3086
Tel: 020 7381 4608
E-mail: info@bhavan.net
www.bhavan.net

Oxford Centre for Hindu Studies
13–15 Magdalen Street
Oxford OX1 3AE
Tel: 01865 304300
E-mail: info@ochs.org.uk
www.ochs.org.uk/index.html

ISKCON Educational Services
Bhaktivedanta ManorDharamMarg
Hilfield Lane
Aldenham
Watford
Herts WD25 8EZ
Tel: 01923 859578
E-mail: ies@iskcon.net
www.iskcon.org.uk/ies/

Temples in the UK

A detailed list of temples in the UK is available from:
www.nchtuk.org/content.php?id=79

Hindu resources on the World Wide Web

Dr Bhavesh Kataria

The Internet is fast becoming the method of choice for most health professionals to gather information about specific issues pertaining to the management of their patients. In this appendix an attempt has been made to present a selection of important and useful websites that may help a healthcare professional in managing a Hindu patient. The sites selected include those specifically dealing with the management of certain medical conditions of high prevalence in the Hindu community. It also includes sites which are of more cultural relevance, providing more in-depth information into the social and cultural identity of Hindus. This allows the healthcare worker to put a given clinical case in a better understood context, which in turn will help to formulate more effective and considered management of the Hindu patient and provide more holistic care.

The amount of information available on the Internet is almost unlimited, and it is continually changing. Rather than providing an exhaustive list of sites, an attempt has been made to include a selection of sites that are thought to be of the most relevance to healthcare professionals. Readers are advised to check the sites from time to time to ensure the information presented remains accurate. The websites were accurate on 12 April 2008.

The sites were obtained by entering a variety of keywords using several search engines. Pre-reviewed sites from the medical press were also evaluated and included. The British Medical Association recommendations were used to assess suitability for inclusion:
- display of most recent information with evidence of regular updates
- display of references and source of information offered

- information about who compiled the site
- site has available contact details
- literal and grammatical accuracy reflecting a well-maintained site
- sites trying to sell products are avoided as far as possible.

Following this, the sites were attributed a star rating from 1 to 5, based on the contents, their relevance and ease of use. Only the higher-rating sites have been included in this appendix.

New information is always being added to the web. The sites included here will hopefully provide enough information to the healthcare worker to enable him or her to provide a comprehensive service to their Hindu patients. It will also provide a taster for the 'seekers' among you to search further in the treasures that Hinduism has to offer.

Website ready reckoner

☆   Not worth wasting time with
☆☆   Some useful material
☆☆☆   Good
☆☆☆☆   Well worth a visit
☆☆☆☆☆   Can't afford to miss this site.

General resources

This section contains sites that are of general importance to the medical community and act as good sources of both general and more directed information.

www.dh.gov.uk (☆☆☆☆)
The Department of Health site has very useful information on a variety of topics related to the care of Hindu patients. Here you can find articles related to the cardiovascular risks of South Asians, the regulations surrounding transplantation of organs from unrelated live donors (which is an issue affecting many Hindus at present) and action against the chewing of betel nuts as well as other topical information.

www.redcross.org.uk (☆☆☆☆)
This is the official site of the Red Cross, providing comprehensive information about its worldwide activities. It can be quite useful to keep abreast of political conflicts and natural disasters in different areas of the world, as some Hindus are migrants from such areas and others may need to travel to these areas.

www.pubmedcentral.nih.gov (☆☆☆☆)
A very easy-to-use site that scans a wide number of medical and life-sciences journals and provides links to full articles in most cases. This site gives access

to articles ranging from the effect of religion and customs in terminal care to detailed molecular biology of illnesses affecting the Hindu population.

Language and communication

www.multikulti.org.uk/ (✩✩✩✩)

This is an excellent site providing information on a variety of health topics in the patient's native language, which can be printed off. The only drawback of this is that only a limited number of languages are represented (currently the only relevant languages for Hindus on this site are Gujarati and Bengali); however, more may be added in future.

www.nhsdirect.nhs.uk/encyclopaedia/ (✩✩✩✩)

This is a very good site, providing accurate and easy-to-access information on a wide range of conditions. There is an easy way to print off patient information leaflets in a wide variety of languages.

www.ethnicityonline.net/default.htm (✩✩✩✩✩)

This is another excellent site. It provides an overview of Hinduism as a whole with a detailed glossary of terms. It also gives more detailed information about the social and cultural issues facing the Hindu patient and the Hindu health worker. The patient information section allows this to be printed in Bengali, which will therefore be extremely useful for this group of Hindus. Unfortunately, this is the only 'Indian' language that the site caters for.

www.library.nhs.uk (✩✩)

This is the National Electronic Library for Health and is a great search tool for a number of topics related to Hindus. It is especially good for printing off a selection of patient information leaflets in a variety of Indian languages (including Gujarati, Hindi, Punjabi, etc.). You have to type the language required in the search box and then select the 'for patients' box. The only downside of this site is the number of layers one has to go through to get to the right information.

www.equip.nhs.uk/language.html (✩✩✩✩)

Although not specifically aimed at Hindu patients, this is an NHS site giving easy access to very useful links. These include details of helplines, support groups and also sites containing information in Hindi, Gujarati, Bengali and other languages.

www.communicate-health.org.uk/card (✩✩✩✩)

Allows you to print off an appointment card in the patient's own language. This ensures that the patient understands when, where and with whom their next appointment is, which in turn improves attendance rates and thus overall patient care.

www.iol.org.uk (☆☆☆)
A useful site to browse if you're looking for an interpreter. It allows you to find one in your area.

www.uktransplant.org.uk/ukt/newsroom/publications/publications.jsp (☆☆☆)
This is the site of the UK Transplant Organisation, promoting organ donation in the Asian community. It has links to leaflets in Hindi, Gujarati and other languages. It also has a useful article about the Hindu religious perspective on organ transplantation.

Healthcare and travel

www.cdc.gov/travel/index.htm (☆☆☆☆☆)
This user-friendly and authoritative site of the Centre for Disease Control and Prevention provides accurate and up-to-date information on the health risks prevalent in specified countries and offers preventative advice. This is particularly important for Hindu pilgrims, who often travel to multiple destinations in India.

www.indmedica.com (☆☆)
This site provides a list of names and contact details of a range of hospitals and nursing homes in India. It also allows a search of physicians according to their speciality. It will be particularly useful in establishing continuing care for patients, who wish to travel to India during their illness.

Medical sites
Mental health issues

www.mind.org.uk (☆☆☆☆)
A very useful site of the leading Mental Health Charity in the UK. It provides useful information to healthcare workers and patients. The site allows access to a range of factsheets dealing with a variety of mental health issues. Some of these are available in the patient's own language (simply type the language in the search box).

www.rethink.org (☆☆☆☆)
This is the website of another mental health charity. It offers details of the Asian Helpline, an information and listening service for any mental health issues, which the patient can access in his/her own language. They also have details of Regional Asian Mental Health Helplines.

www.aquarius.org.uk (☆☆☆)
This site has details for the Birmingham Asian Alcohol Service, which provides counselling and information in the patient's native language.

Cardiology

www.bhf.org.uk (☆☆☆☆)

This is the site of the British Heart Foundation and provides very useful information on the cardiac issues facing the Indian population. The factfile titled 'South Asians and Heart Disease' is particularly useful and provides details on the Asian Quitline.

www.epi.bris.ac.uk (☆☆☆☆)

This provides a cardiovascular disease (CVD) risk calculator adjusted for minority ethnic groups (type 'cvd risk' in the search box). It should be used in conjunction with the current CVD risk calculators issued by the Joint Societies as it is pending full validation.

www.bcs.com and www.bcpa.co.uk are the sites of the British Cardiac Society and the British Cardiac Patients Association. The BCS provides more in-depth information about cardiac issues affecting the Asian community. The BCPA gives access to many useful patient information leaflets.

Diabetes

www.diabetes.org.uk/home.htm (☆☆☆☆☆)

This is the leading diabetes charity in the UK. The site is excellent as it provides a wide range of practical information about diabetes to patients. The site can be viewed in a number of different languages. The association also has a telephone helpline providing information and support in the patient's own language.

Thalassaemia

www.ukts.org (☆☆☆☆)

This is the website of the UK Thalassaemia Association. The site provides very easy-to-read information about the different types of thalassaemias, which can be printed and given to patients. It also has simple clinical information regarding diagnosis and management. It has very useful links to a number of sites worldwide.

www.thalassaemia.org.cy (☆☆☆☆☆)

This is an excellent and well-designed site dealing with everything you ever wanted to know about thalassaemia and more. There are very good diagrams describing the genetics, which are handy when explaining the condition to patients. There are also a number of books available (free to download) with more detailed specialist information about all aspects, ranging from diagnosis to psychological issues arising in the patient and the family.

Osteoporosis

www.nos.org.uk/healthprof.asp (★★★★☆)

The healthcare section of the National Osteoporosis Society is very easy to navigate and provides access to a wide selection of patient information leaflets as well as general information and local support groups for patients with osteoporosis.

Cultural aspects of Hinduism

The aim of this section is to provide the practitioner with web resources that deal more with the cultural aspects of Hinduism, the religion, the philosophy and values that Hindus live by as well as other important aspects of Hindu life.

Ayurveda

Ayurveda literally means 'the science of living'. In its original form, it is a holistic system of medicine and lifestyle practised for more than 5000 years. The sites below provide a comprehensive overview. Another site is included under the 'Religion and Philosophy' section.

www.allayurveda.com/discover.htm (★★★★☆)

This site contains everything about Ayurveda that you ever wanted to know. It is very easy to understand and hence a good starting point for the novice. The site is very practically arranged and so getting the relevant information is easy.

www.ayurvedic.org (★★★★☆)

This is another great site with access to all aspects of Ayurvedic medicine. This site has an online consultation facility, which allows the health professional to communicate directly with a qualified Ayurvedic practitioner regarding any treatment his/her patient may be using. The glossary of common Ayurvedic herbs is well organised and comprehensive (go to 'Ayruveda', 'About Ayurveda', 'Herbs'). The site also allows one to find out one's physical and psychological constitution, which forms the basis of treatment in Ayurveda, thus providing the health professional with a fuller understanding of the type of treatments their patients may be using (go to 'Ayurveda', 'Check your VPK').

Vegetarianism

Hindus are traditionally vegetarians, with the firm belief that the killing of animals for sense pleasure is sinful. Milk products and its derivatives are allowed, provided no harm is caused to the animals in the process.

www.vegsoc.org/info/index.html (★★★★★)
This is the official website of the Vegetarian Society of the UK. It is very well organised and user-friendly. Traditionally, many Hindus are vegetarian and most have milk and milk products. Many ailments in the Hindu population arise from dietary deficiencies, such as iron, zinc, vitamin B12, calcium, etc. This site provides the healthcare professional with very good references to nutritional requirements and provides valuable information on sources of essential nutrients, daily requirements and even suggestions of meal plans.

www.bda.uk.com/Downloads/vegetarianfoodfacts.pdf (★★★)
This is a patient information leaflet detailing a number of nutritional issues affecting the vegetarian.

The British Dietetic Association (www.bda.uk.com/sgroupspublic.html) also has a subgroup called the Multicultural Nutrition Group. They can provide useful leaflets about healthy eating specific to Asian vegetarians. Contact 0121 2008080. The above site has email contacts for further information.

Religion and philosophy

http://hinduism.iskcon.com (★★★★★)
A superb website on Hinduism. It deals with all aspects of Hinduism, both philosophical and cultural, in a very comprehensive way, using illustrations and diagrams to clarify some complex concepts. It is very user-friendly and easy to navigate to the areas of interest. A must for those interested in understanding Hinduism well.

www.bvashram.org/categories/Questions-and-Answers (★★★★★)
A very good site, from a prominent Vaishnava tradition, addressing the main concepts of Hinduism in a Q & A format. Very easy to understand and a good source of information for both novice and practising Hindus.

www.nchtuk.org/index.php (★★★★★)
This is the official site of the National Council of Hindu Temples, the largest umbrella organisation representing Hindus in the UK. The site contains current affairs affecting Hindus as well as very useful and clear overviews of Hinduism and its core beliefs. A variety of resources are available. The section on Ayurveda provides a good overview of the basic principles of this site.

www.hinduism.co.za (★★★★)
A great website with very easy and comprehensive links arranged in topical fashion dealing with all aspects of Hindu lifestyle and practices. The scientific links provide an overview of the history of Ayurveda and links dealing with Ayurveda in much more detail.

Scriptures

Hinduism is based on the teachings of the four Vedas. These are ancient texts written in Sanskrit. The essential teachings of the Vedas have been explained in the main scriptures of Hinduism, which are the Bhagavad-Gita (part of the Mahabharat), Srimad Bhagavatam and the Ramayana.

www.prabhupadavani.org (☆☆☆☆☆)
This is an excellent website, providing access to some of the most important Hindu scriptures, the Bhagavad-Gita and the Srimad Bhagavatam. The Gita provides the philosophical foundation of Hinduism as spoken by the Supreme Personality of Godhead, Lord Krishna Himself. The Bhagavatam details the life and teachings of the great saints of India and includes the history of Lord Krishna. These scriptures can be either read as a direct translation or as a Sanskrit transliteration of the original text with an elaborate and scholarly explanation of each verse by HDG AC Bhaktivedanta Swami Prabhupada, one of the most prominent saints in recent times. There is also access to more detailed lectures and discourses on these scriptures by the author providing a more in-depth understanding of the philosophy and its practical application in daily life.

www.valmikiramayan.net (☆☆☆☆)
This is a site providing direct access to the whole text of the Ramayana. It is interspersed with quite detailed information and dissection of the original verses, making it difficult to follow the prose of the story itself.

APPENDIX 5

Dietary leaflets

Aude Cholet

These diet sheets have been adapted with help from the Nutrition and Dietetic departments of:

- Hillingdon Hospital NHS Trust, Hillingdon Hospital, Pield Heath Road, Uxbridge UB8 3NN
- The North West London Hospitals NHS Trust, Northwick Park Hospital, Watford Road, Harrow, Middlesex, HA1 3UJ.

The Hindu vegetarian diet has been discussed in Chapter 3. Due to the specific needs of a lacto-vegetarian diet the following diet sheets have been designed to help treat patients in this group (diet sheets 1–4). Chapter 2 shows most Hindus are of Indian descent and are a group more prone to vascular disease and diabetes. Diet sheets 5–8 look at this in context of the dietary needs:

1 Dietary advice for low calcium
2 Dietary advice for low vitamin D
3 Dietary advice for low iron
4 Dietary advice for low vitamin B12
5 Healthy eating for diabetic patients
6 Healthy eating to lose weight
7 Healthy eating for patients with high cholesterol/heart problems
8 Table of food choice – attached to diet sheets 5, 6 and 7.

1 Dietary advice for low calcium

Calcium is a mineral vital for strong teeth and bones and in small amounts is involved in muscle contraction and processes such as blood clotting. New bone is being made and old bone lost all the time. An adult replaces his/her skeleton every 10 years and a child every two years.

Make sure you care for your bones

- Enjoy a varied balanced diet.
- Try to include dairy foods in your diet. Choose low fat varieties if weight is a problem.
- Get plenty of weight-bearing exercise.

TABLE 1 Sources of calcium

FOOD	CALCIUM (MG)
200 ml full cream milk	225
200 ml semi-skimmed milk	240
200 ml skimmed milk	244
25 g cheddar cheese	185
100 g cottage cheese	127
100 g ice-cream	100
100 g yoghurt	140
2 large slices of bread	100
100 g baked beans	53
50 g almonds	120
50 g hazel/brazil nuts	80
100 g boiled spinach/kale	160
100 g fresh apricots	73
100 g figs	250
100 g fresh orange	50

(Milk: 200 ml = 1/3 pint; 25 grams = 1 ounce)

TABLE 2 How much calcium do we need?

AGE GROUP	CALCIUM NEEDED PER DAY (MG)
1–3 years	350
4–6 years	450
7–10 years	550
11–18 years	800–1000
Adults	700–1000
Post menopausal women	1500

Try to include at least three items from the following each day:

- ⅓ pint (200 ml) milk (whole, semi skimmed or skimmed).
- 4 oz (100 g) small carton or 7 tablespoons of yoghurt.
- 1–1½ slices (30–40 g) of hard cheese, e.g. cheddar cheese.
- ⅓ pint (200 ml) fortified soya milk (i.e. soya milk with added calcium).

Calcium deficiency

A deficiency of calcium leads to weak bones and teeth causing osteoporosis. We lose calcium naturally from our bones, as we get older. Weak bones are prone to fracture.

Those at risk

Women approaching the menopause have hormone changes, which tend to accelerate bone density loss. Those Hindu patients with a low intake of dairy products, and poor exercise levels, especially the elderly will be more at risk.

What to do?

Plenty of calcium in the diet of young people helps to build large reservoirs, which consequently takes longer to deplete as they get older. Fractures are then less likely.

And finally

- As you can see milk and milk products are the best sources of calcium.
- Some people are unable to take milk. If this is so choose soya milk that has had calcium added.
- Vitamin D is important for calcium to be absorbed from our food.
- Regular exposure to sunlight provides vitamin D since it can be produced just under the skin. Good food sources include margarines and spreads, some fortified breakfast cereals. Some bread and chapattis may also be fortified with this.
- Only full-fat diary products contain significant levels of vitamin D.

2 Dietary advice for low vitamin D
What is vitamin D?

It is a fat-soluble vitamin essential for helping the body to absorb calcium from food and deposit it into the bones.

Sources of vitamin D

Most vitamin D is derived from exposure of the skin to sunlight. There are only a few good dietary sources; these include butter, margarine and fortified breakfast cereals.

Deficiency

This may occur in people who are not regularly exposed to the sun. Severe deficiency causes rickets in children and osteomalacia in adults. The bones do not take up calcium properly and they become weak, causing a deformed skeleton and bone pain.

Those at risk of deficiency

Young children, vegetarians, and those wearing dark thick clothing or who live in urban areas out of the sun; women who have had multiple pregnancies and people who are housebound.

Note: very high levels of vitamin D are rare unless you take excessive vitamin D supplements such as cod liver oil supplements. Always ensure you follow the recommended guidelines.

Ideas to help you

- Aim to go outside every day in sunny weather. Wear loose thin clothing. Long periods of sunbathing are *not* recommended.
- If you are unable to go out, dietary sources of vitamin D are important. These include:
  - Paneer, yogurt, lassi, fortified margarines, spreads and butter ghee (but not vegetable ghee).
  - Evaporated or condensed milk (try on fruit as a dessert).
  - Cheese – full-fat varieties have most vitamin D.

Many people nowadays are advised to take less fat in their diet. Vitamin D is only found in animal (including dairy) fats. If you are unable to go out in the sun and are not able to take the foods recommended above, please ask to see a dietician.

Exercise

Exercise every day, as it promotes calcium deposition in bones.

3 Dietary advice for low iron

Iron is a mineral. Its main role is as an oxygen carrier in the blood. It is essential for healthy blood formation.

Deficiency

A lack of iron in the diet causes **anaemia**. This means you have reduced ability to transport oxygen around the body, which results in breathlessness, fatigue and pallor.

Causes of iron deficiency

Excessive blood loss is the main cause of anaemia, often made worse by a poor iron intake.

People at risk of deficiency

Menstruating and pregnant women (especially those who do not eat red meat); the elderly and frail with poor appetites; growing children, especially those who are fussy eaters and who avoid red meat.

Very high intakes are rare unless there is excessive use of iron supplements.

Sources of iron

Dietary iron exists in two forms:

- **Haem-iron,** which is found in red meats (and offal).
- **Non-haem iron,** which is found in wholegrain cereals, beans, lentils and nuts.

Note: To absorb non-haem iron it is vital to take a food high in vitamin C, e.g. orange or vegetable juice at the same meal.

Examples of sources of non-haem-iron

- Bread, especially chapattis and other wholemeal, malt, granary and fortified breads.
- Iron-fortified breakfast cereals, e.g. Branflakes, Allbran or Ready brek. All breakfast cereals containing iron will state the nutritional information on the pack.
- Dark green leafy vegetables, e.g. spinach, broccoli, kale.
- Pulses: lentils, peas, baked beans, kidney beans, chickpeas, tofu, hummus.
- Dried fruit: figs, apricots, prunes, sultanas, raisins.
- Nuts and seeds, e.g. almonds, brazil nuts, hazelnuts, cashews, peanuts, tahini paste, sunflower seeds.
- Also: treacle, cocoa, plain chocolate, Bovril, Oxo, Marmite, curry powder and liquorice.

Sources of vitamin C

Always take *with* the meal to help absorb non-haem iron from food. Vitamin C is found mainly in fresh fruit and vegetables. Vitamin C is lost during cooking, so do not boil vegetables for too long and avoid reheating where possible. Vitamin C levels fall over time and so vegetables should be eaten when fresh. Vitamin C is found in green vegetables such as broccoli, cabbage, green and red peppers, karela, sprouts, peas, kale, tomatoes and root vegetables such as potatoes and carrots. It is also found in fresh fruits such as guava, mango, kiwifruit, pawpaw, strawberries, raspberries, oranges, grapefruits and blackcurrants; also in lemon juice and blackcurrant juice.

Tea

Tea contains a substance called tannin that can reduce the body's ability to absorb iron from food, so avoid drinking tea with food. Wait at least 1 hour after eating. It may be better to drink a glass of fruit juice or blackcurrant squash at meal times instead, as these drinks contain high quantities of vitamin C. Alternatively, use weak teas or even herbal teas if you wish.

4 Dietary advice for low vitamin B12

Vitamin B12 (also known as B_{12}) is present in foods of animal origin such as meat, fish and dairy foods. It is needed to prevent anaemia.

For vegetarians, milk is an important source of this vitamin. Heating milk will reduce some of the B12.

Other foods that contain B12 are cheese and yogurt. Some breakfast cereals are also fortified with vitamin B12. Check the label.

In addition, good sources include yeast extracts such as Marmite, Bovril, Tastex and Barmene, which can be spread on bread, added to soups or taken directly (1–2 teaspoons a day).

5 Healthy eating for diabetic patients

(Diabetes UK has published a 10 steps guideline to eating well for people with diabetes.)

1 Eat three regular meals

It is important to eat three meals a day without snacking on high calorie foods such as chevra or ghatia. This will help regulate your blood sugars and appetite.

2 At each meal include starchy carbohydrate foods, preferably high fibre (slowly absorbed)

Wholegrain breads and chapattis (without added fat), unsweetened wholegrain breakfast cereals, basmati rice, pasta and fresh potatoes/sweet potatoes are all healthy foods and can be eaten in limited amounts. Try to use medium brown flour in cooking. Choose 6–8 portions from the following group daily.

- 1 slice wholegrain bread from large medium cut loaf.
- 2 small thin cut slices wholegrain bread.
- 3 oz (1 teacup) boiled basmati rice or pasta.
- 1 medium-sized thin medium brown chapatti or rotlo (no fat added).
- ½ medium-sized baked bhakris (no fat added).
- 1 small naan (no fat added, wholemeal if possible).

- 1 small rotlo.
- 2 small egg-size (sweet) potatoes (mashed or boiled) *or* 1 medium-sized jacket potato.
- 1 oz (30 g) or 5 tablespoons wholegrain breakfast cereal.
- 3 wholegrain crispbreads.
- 2 plain biscuits (rich tea, malted, nice).

3 Cut down on fat, particularly saturated fat and choose monounsaturated fat instead

Cut out butter, ghee and coconut cream. Avoid condensed/evaporated milk and foods that have been prepared with it (e.g. barfi). Use semi-skimmed milk and make/buy low fat yoghurt. Use semi-skimmed milk and/or low fat yoghurt in cooking or for lassi/paneer.

If you need to lose weight, use only small amounts of cooking oil (1 teaspoon per person per dish) and soft margarines that are high in monounsaturated fats. Read labels on packaged foods and aim for foods with 5 g of fat (or less) per 100 g of food.

4 Eat more fruit and vegetables, aim for at least five servings a day

These are low in calories, high in fibre and protective vitamins. Aim for maximum 3 pieces of fruit per day (1 medium-sized piece of fruit or 1 handful at a time) and **at least** 2 portions/handful of vegetables per day. It is a good idea to have a mixture of cooked *and* raw vegetables every day (e.g. bhindi/brinjal in curry *and* tomato/cucumber salad). (Note: potato is *not* counted as a vegetable.)

5 Include more beans and lentils (dhals)

Beans and pulses (all dhals) are high in fibre and low in fat. They also provide good food value when eaten with bread, chapattis, rice, pasta and other cereals. You should eat some **daily**.

Here are some ideas:

- Bean or lentil curry with rice (with extra vegetables/salad).
- Dhal and chapatti (with extra vegetables/salad).
- Baked beans on toast (with extra vegetables/salad).
- Lentil sauce with spaghetti/pasta (with extra vegetables/salad).

6 Limit sugar and sugary foods

Avoid sugar and sugary foods and drinks. If you wish, you can use an artificial sweetener in tablet, powder or liquid form, e.g. Canderel, Hermesetes, Sweetex. Some recipes can be modified to use sweeteners instead of sugar.

7 Reduce salt to 6 g (1 heaped teaspoon) or less per day

Avoid salt in cooking and at the table as well as salty snacks (salted nuts, *sev*, *ganthia* etc.). Salt is naturally present in most foods so you don't have to add extra salt.

8 Drink alcohol in moderation only

If you drink alcohol, have a maximum 2 units per day for women and 3 for men. Ask your health professional for more advice. (Many Hindus do not drink.)

9 Diabetic foods or drinks offer no benefit

Avoid buying 'diabetic' products as they are more expensive and can be high in fat. Diabetic needs to eat a healthy diet, not a 'diabetic' diet.

10 Finally, get on the move!

Exercise, as well as diet, will help you lose weight, control your blood sugar levels and lower your cholesterol levels. As little as 30 minutes per of moderate activity (walking, stairs, housework, cycling, gardening etc.) will have beneficial effect (however, you need to feel your heart beating faster). You can choose to do 30 minutes or twice 15 minutes to fit in with your life.

6 Healthy eating to lose weight

Slimming sensibly means achieving a healthy weight through eating a variety of wholesome foods. This will help you to keep your weight, blood sugars and cholesterol under control.

Here are some helpful hints:

1 Eat regular meals

It is important to eat three meals a day without snacking on high calorie foods such as chevra or ghatia.

2 Cut down on fat

Cut out butter and ghee. Use only small amounts of cooking oil (1 teaspoon per person per dish) and soft margarines that are high in monounsaturated fats. Read labels on packaged foods and aim for foods with 5 g of fat (or less) per 100 g of food.

3 Select your starchy foods

Wholegrain breads, chapattis (without added fat), unsweetened wholegrain breakfast cereals, basmati rice, pasta and fresh potatoes are all healthy foods and can be eaten in limited amounts. Try to use medium brown flour in cooking. Choose 6–8 portions from the following groups daily.

- 1 slice wholegrain bread from large medium cut loaf.
- 2 small thin cut slices of wholegrain bread.
- 3 oz (1 teacup) boiled basmati rice or pasta.
- 1 medium-sized thin brown chapatti or rotlo (no fat added).
- ½ medium-sized baked bhakris (no fat added).
- 1 small naan (no fat added).
- 1 small rotlo.
- 2 small egg-size (sweet) potatoes (mashed or boiled) *or* 1 medium-sized jacket potato.
- 1 oz (30 g) or 5 tablespoons wholegrain breakfast cereal.
- 3 wholegrain crispbreads.
- 2 plain biscuits (rich tea, malted, nice).

4 Give up sugar

Avoid sugar and sugary foods and drinks. If you wish, you can use an artificial sweetener in tablet, powder or liquid form, e.g. Canderel, Hermesetes, Sweetex. Most recipes can be modified to use sweeteners instead of sugar.

5 Fill up on vegetables and salads

These are low in calories, high in fibre and protective vitamins. Try and eat with every meal.

6 Don't forget the protein foods

Beans and pulses provide good food value when eaten with bread, chapattis, rice, pasta and other cereals. You should eat some daily. They are also high in fibre and low in fat.

Here are some ideas:

- Bean or lentil curry with rice (with extra vegetables/salad).
- Dhal and chapatti (with extra vegetables/salad).
- Baked beans on toast (with extra vegetables/salad).
- Lentil sauce with spaghetti/pasta (with extra vegetables/salad).

7 Keep to low calorie desserts

Choose fresh fruit, low fat plain yogurt or virtually fat free fruit yogurt.

8 Be wise with your drinks

Lassi can be prepared with a low fat yogurt. An artificial sweetener should be used instead of sugar.

Choose low calorie drinks such as water, diet fizzy drinks, low calorie squashes.

If you drink, keep alcohol to a minimum.

9 Get on the move

Exercise, as well as diet, will help you lose weight, control your blood sugar levels and lower your cholesterol levels. As little as 30 minutes per of moderate activity (walking, stairs, housework, cycling, gardening etc.) will have beneficial effect. You can choose to do 30 minutes or twice 15 minutes to fit in with your life.

10 Weekly weight

Weigh yourself once a week in the same clothes and at the same time of day. Set yourself a realistic target: losing more than 1 or 2 lb (450g or 900g) a week is not likely to lead to long term weight loss.

7 Healthy eating for patients with high cholesterol/heart problems

The British Heart Foundation has published a seven steps guideline to eating well for people with high cholesterol and/or at risk of developing heart problems.

1 Eat more fruit and vegetables, aim for at least 5 servings a day

These are low in calories, high in fibre and protective vitamins. Aim for 3 pieces of fruit per day and **at least** 2 portions/handful of vegetables per day. It is a good idea to have a mixture of cooked *and* raw vegetables every day (e.g. bhindi/brinjal in curry *and* tomato/cucumber salad). (Note: potato is *not* counted as a vegetable.)

2 Cut down on fat, particularly saturated fat and choose monounsaturated fat instead

- Cut out butter, ghee and coconut cream. Avoid condensed/evaporated milk and foods that have been prepared with it (e.g. barfi).
- Use semi-skimmed milk and make/buy low fat yogurt. Use semi-skimmed milk and/or low fat yogurt in cooking or for lassi/paneer.
- If you need to lose weight, use only small amounts of cooking oil (1 teaspoon per person per dish) and soft margarines that are high in monounsaturated fats.

࣫ Beware of hidden fats so read labels on packaged foods and aim for foods with 10g of fat (or less) per 100g of food.

3 Aim for at least 2 portions of oily fish a week

This is to increase intake of omega-3 fats: these fats are protective against heart problems. However, this is not possible when you are vegetarian. You can discuss the benefits/disadvantages of vegetarian omega-3 supplements with your health professional.

4 Keep a healthy weight

It is especially important to lose weight if you carry most of it around your waist (i.e. near the heart). Ask your health professional to check your waist circumference to find out if you need to reduce your waist size.

To help with losing weight, it is important to eat three meals a day without snacking on high calorie foods such as chevra or ghatia. This will help regulate your metabolism and appetite. Increasing your physical activity is also vital (*see* point 11).

5 Reduce salt to 6g (1 heaped teaspoon) or less per day

Avoid salt in cooking and at the table as well as salty snacks (salted nuts, *sev*, *ganthia* etc.). Salt is naturally present in most foods so you don't have to add extra salt.

If you buy packaged foods (sandwiches, cereals etc.), check the label: you should avoid foods that contain 1.25g or more of salt per 100g of food (same as 0.5g of sodium/100g).

6 Drink alcohol within sensible limits

Some Hindus do not drink alcohol. For those who do, a maximum of 2 units per day for women and 3 for men is recommended. Ask your health professional for more advice if needed.

7 Don't forget beans and lentils (dhal)

Beans and pulses (all dhal) are high in fibre and low in fat. They can also help decrease cholesterol levels. You should eat some **daily**.

Here are some ideas:
࣫ Bean or lentil curry with rice (with extra vegetables/salad).
࣫ Dhal and chapatti (with extra vegetables/salad).
࣫ Baked beans on toast (with extra vegetables/salad).
࣫ Lentil sauce with spaghetti/pasta (with extra vegetables/salad).

Finally, get on the move!

Exercise, as well as diet, will help you lose weight, control your blood sugar levels and lower your cholesterol levels. As little as 30 minutes per of moderate activity (walking, stairs, housework, cycling, gardening etc.) will have beneficial effect (however, you need to feel your heart beating faster). You can choose to do 30 minutes or twice 15 minutes to fit in with your life.

FOODS	CHOOSE THESE	INSTEAD OF THESE
Bread and other cereals Keep to the amounts listed in point 3 on page 109	Wholemeal breads, rolls, baked bhakris and naan. Unsweetened wholegrain breakfast cereal and muesli, porridge oats. Potato/sweet potatoes in their skins – boiled or 'jacket'. Rice, pasta and mogo. Toasted or microwaved papdi or papad.	Croissants, savoury cheese biscuits, cream crackers, puff pastry biscuits. Sweetened cereals and crunchy muesli, seero. Puri, paratha, thepla, dhebra, andhwo bateta pawa, dhokra, dhokri. Crisps, fried Indian snacks, e.g. sev, ganthia, chevdo etc. Bhajjia, samosa, chips, mogo chips. Fries, chips, roast potatoes.
Vegetables and salads	All fresh and frozen vegetables. Eat with every meal.	Deep fried vegetables, e.g. mushrooms, vegetable bhajjias, patra bhajjia.
Fruit	Fresh fruit or tinned fruit in natural juice – 3 portions (3 handfuls) a day (including fresh, unsweetened mango pulp). Dried food: 1 tablespoon = one portion.	Sweetened fruit juice, tinned fruit in syrup and tinned mango pulp.
Pulses and lentils Eat daily	Cooked mung, masur, toor, chora, urad, channa pigeon peas, baked beans and soya beans cooked in very little oil.	Bean and lentil curries with oily or creamy sauces. Deep fried channa, mung and dhal snacks.
Nuts	Unsalted nuts and seeds, **1 level tablespoon per day maximum.**	Salted nuts, coconut.
Milk, yoghurts and milk-based desserts	1 pint (600 ml) skimmed milk or semi-skimmed milk or calcium enriched soya milk per day. 1 carton plain unsweetened low fat yoghurt or virtually fat free fruit yoghurt, e.g. Diet Ski or Shape, may be taken instead of ¼ pint (150 ml) skimmed milk.	Full fat milk (red top and silver top). Cream, fruit yoghurts, ice-cream, whipped topping, coffee whitener, condensed and evaporated milk. Shrikand, doodh pak, gulab jamun, penda, ras malai and kulfi, and other desserts made with full fat milk, yoghurt and milk powder. Sweetened soya milk.

continued.

FOODS	CHOOSE THESE	INSTEAD OF THESE
Cheese	1 small tub skimmed milk cheese, e.g. cottage cheese, curd cheese or unsweetened fromage frais. Paneer made with semi-skimmed milk. 2 oz/week: Edam, Camembert, blue type and reduced fat hard cheeses.	Hard cheese, cream cheese, full fat cheese spread, paneer made from full fat milk.
Fats Watch the amount	Monounsaturated fats, e.g. olive oil, olive spread, rapeseed oil, avocado oil.	Margarine, low fat spread or cooking oil high in polyunsaturated fat, e.g. corn or sunflower oil, butter, coconut oil, blended vegetable oil, ghee, mayonnaise, fatty sauces and salad creams and dressings, pastries and deep fried foods.
Sweets, preserves, spreads	Artificial sweeteners, e.g. Sweetex, Hermesetas or Canderel. Pickles in vinegar and lime juice. Herbs and spices, Oxo cubes, Bovril, vegetable stock cubes, salt, pepper. Sugar free jelly.	Sugar. Gor, sakar, peanut butter, jam, honey, marmalades. Pickles and chutneys in oil and sugar/gor. Chocolates, sweets, ice lollies, jellies, instant desserts and mousses. All Indian sweets, e.g. jalebi, halwa, barfi, etc.
Biscuits, cakes and made-up sauces	1 plain biscuit a day if desired, e.g. Rich Tea or Marie.	Sweet biscuits (e.g. chocolate, cream-filled), pastry, pies, cakes, rich sauces.
Drinks	Tea (between meals), coffee, mineral water, low calorie drinks, e.g. diet fizzy drinks, sugar-free squashes. Lassi (made with low fat yogurt and no sugar).	Sugary drinks, e.g. Vimto, Ribena, Lucozade and fizzy drinks. Full fat yoghurt lassi, hot chocolate, malted milk drinks. Alcohol including low sugar beers.

Glossary

Nima Suchak

agyarasa   *See* ekadashi.

ahimsa   Non-violence, an important Hindu principle, practiced by Mahatma Gandhi.

Anna Prashana Samskara   Weaning ceremony for a baby, when the child is first given grains at five or six months.

antaryami   'The Lord within', a term referring to a form of God within the heart. According to Hindu theology, God is found in three places: (1) everywhere (2) within the heart, and (3) without, far beyond this world.

Antyeshti Samskara   Funeral rites; the rites taking place immediately after death.

ashrama   'Place of spiritual shelter' or 'hermitage'; it also refers to each of the four traditional stages of life (implying that each stage is intended for spiritual growth).

atman   The atman ('real self' or soul) resides in all living creatures, as the source of life and awareness.

aum   *See* om.

Ayurveda	The medical science enunciated within the sacred Veda. Also the text itself, which is, specifically, one of the four 'Upavedas'.
ben	Sister; often added as a suffix to first name, e.g. 'Sarojben', 'Lakshmiben', etc.
Bhagavad-Gita	The teachings on spiritual life and devotion to God spoken by the Lord Krishna to his friend Arjuna just before the great battle of Kurukshetra. The *Bhagavad-Gita* is part of the *Mahabharata.*
bhagavan	The most popular term for God (when conceived of as a person). It means 'one who possesses unlimited opulence'. These 'opulent qualities' have been listed as strength, wealth, fame, beauty, knowledge and renunciation.
bhai/bhaiya	Brother; often added as a suffix to first name, e.g. 'Rameshbhai'.
bindi	A red dot worn on the forehead by Hindu women, traditionally signifying wedded status. It has today become a fashion accessory, even for single women.
brahman	Spirit (as differentiated from matter); the Supreme (or God) in his impersonal, all-pervasive aspect.
brahmin	A member of one of the four classes (varnas) in the varnashrama social system, typically involved in teaching, preaching and priestly activities.
chandan	Sandalwood, particularly in its form as a cooling paste. It is sometimes used in forming tilak (*see* tilak).
Cuda Karana Samskara	Ceremony for the first shaving of the hair of a child.
darshana	Literally 'seeing'; taking audience of the temple deity or a holy person.
darshanas	'perspective'; refers to each of the six orthodox schools of thought; often called 'the six darshanas'.
dharma	Loosely translated as 'religious principles', or 'individual duty'. More precisely, dharma means 'duties that sustain us according to our natural

disposition'. There are two main classifications: sanatana (eternal) dharma and varnashrama dharma.

Dharma-Shastra The scriptures, supplementary to the *Vedas*, which consist of ethical, domestic, social and governmental laws for practising Hindus.

dhoti A single long piece of cloth, usually of cotton or silk, which is the standard garment worn on the lower part of the body by orthodox Hindu men.

didi Affectionate term for an older sister.

dosha Similar to the archaic 'humour'; an intrinsic factor of the body and mind which may become excited and imbalanced, either conferring a disposition to, or actually causing, morbidities. The three primary doshas are combinations of the five elements. Vata is considered to be a combination of ether and space; pitta, a combination of fire and water; and kapha is composed of water and earth elements.

dukanwala Shopkeeper.

dvija A member of one of the three classes (*brahmanins*, *kshatriyas*, and *vaishyas*) who are 'twice-born' by dint of initiation by a spiritual master/guru. The term is most often used in reference to *brahmanins*.

ekadashi A day on which Vaishnavas fast from grains and beans and increase their remembrance of Vishnu, or one of his forms such as Rama and Krishna. It falls on the eleventh day of both the waxing and waning moons, and is also known as agyarasa.

Ganesh One of the most popular Hindu deities, depicted with an elephant's head. He is the son of Shiva and Parvati, and the lord of beginnings and entrance ways.

Ganges water Water from the river flowing from the peaks of the Himalayas to the Bay of Bengal. Hindus consider that anyone who comes into contact with Ganges water is delivered from sin and thus liberated.

Garbhadhana Samskara A Vedic purificatory process performed by couples for the conception of children.

Gayatri mantra	One of the most important Hindi prayers, traditionally chanted thrice daily by brahmins.
Grihya Sutras	A section of the Vedas outlining the rites of passage called samskaras.
guna	Literally 'rope', it often refers to the three qualities or 'modes' of material nature: *sattva-guna* (goodness), *rajo-guna* (passion), and *tamo-guna* (ignorance).
guru	A spiritual master who initiates and instructs people about self-realisation and God consciousness; also used as a term of respect for any teacher.
Gurudev	Title of respect given to one's spiritual master.
ISKCON	The International Society for Krishna Consciousness, often called the Hare Krishna movement. It is a strand of Bengali Vaishnavism, which follows the devotional saint Chaitanya (1486–1534), and is well known for its sari-clad and saffron-clothed Western followers.
janoi	The sacred thread; a loop of three to nine threads draped over the left shoulder and torso of a male *brahmin*, used while chanting mantras.
japa	The quiet or silent chanting of a mantra, usually performed individually.
japa mala	Beads used during japa meditation; usually 108 in number.
Jatakarma Samskara	Birth ceremony to welcome a newborn child.
jati	Community or occupational group within Hinduism. Jati are usually considered sub-categories of the four varnas (main social classifications).
jyotisha	'The science of light'; a Vedic astrology system still prevalent amongst many Hindus and intimately linked to ideas of reincarnation and karma.
kajol	A black dot applied to a child's forehead and intended to divert the attention of strangers from

the baby's eyes, thus avoiding envy and other negative influences.

kanthi mala   Sacred beads worn around the neck, especially by Vaishnava devotees.

kapha   In Ayurvedic medicine, the force or humour symbolised by earth and water.

karma   Literally 'action'; it also refers to 'reaction' and the accumulation of such reactions, as in the popular idioms 'good karma' and 'bad karma'; it alludes to the universal law of individual accountability (i.e. 'the law of karma').

Karnavedha Samskara   Ceremony for piercing the ears of an infant.

kavacha   Talisman; a sacred charm worn for protection.

Krishna   One of the most popular Hindu deities, a form of Vishnu, often considered as Supreme Godhead by Vaishnavas, and many Hindus in the UK. Some groups consider Krishna the source of all incarnations.

kumkum   A red cosmetic powder, used in making bindi.

kurta   A traditional Indian loose-fitting shirt.

maa   'Mother', usually used as an affectionate form of address; shortened form of 'mata'.

Mahabharata   One of the most important Hindus epics. A poem describing a period of Hindu history (traditionally, around 3000 BC). It includes the Bhagavad-Gita, one of the most important contemporary religious texts.

maha-mantra   'The great mantra'. A chant widely popularised in India by the 16th century saint Chaitanya, and later throughout the world by ISKCON. It reads: 'Hare Krishna, Hare Krishna, Krishna Krishna, Hare Hare/Hare Rama, Hare Rama, Rama Rama, Hare Hare'.

maha-prasada   Consecrated food taken directly from the shrine after it has been offered to the sacred image; considered to bestow immense spiritual benefit (*see also* prasada).

maharaja	'Great ruler'; a term of address to kings and sannyasis (monks).
mangala sutra	An auspicious necklace, often of black and gold beads, constantly worn by a wife to symbolise her righteous marriage.
mantra	Literally, 'that which delivers the mind' a string of sacred syllables chanted repetitively to purify the mind and fix it on the divine.
marg	'Path'; it usually refers to one of the specific yogas, or 'ways of linking to the divine'. Books usually list three or four main paths, or types of yoga.
masi/kaki	'Aunt'; masi is the mother's sister; kaki is the wife of the father's younger brother. Both can be used as a suffix to address Hindu women; for example Bhanu becomes 'Bhanumasi' or 'Bhanukaki'.
mataji	'Respected mother'; a term of address for a Hindu woman other than one's wife; also a respectful term of address for Shakti, the Goddess.
moksha/mukti	Liberation from the cycle of birth and death.
murti	'Form', usually referring to a sacred image of God or a particular deity.
Nama Karana Samskara	Name-giving ceremony performed on (or around) the tenth day after a child's birth.
Niskramana Samskara	First outing ceremony for a new baby.
om	(also **aum**) The most important mantra (sacred syllable) in Hinduism.
paramatma	'The Supreme Soul' (God) or sometimes translated as 'the Super Soul', referring to God within the heart (*see* 'Antaryami'.)
pitta	In Ayurvedic medicine, the force or humour symbolised by fire.
prabhu	A respectful form of address, meaning 'master'.
prakriti	Matter; the non-conscious, transient elements of God's creation; it includes the physical body and the mind, distinct from the eternal atman (self).

prasada	Literally, 'mercy' or 'grace'; usually refers to sanctified food that has been offered to God; may include other things previously used in worship, such as water, flowers and incense.
puja	Worship; particularly refers to the daily, ritualistic adoration of the murti (sacred image) within the temple.
pujari	A devotee who performs the puja, direct worship and service to the temple deity.
Puranas	The sections of Hindu literature consisting of stories.
Pushti Marg	A Hindu tradition that originated with the devotional revivalist Vallabha (1479–1531). Its followers place much emphasis on home worship, especially of Krishna in his form as an infant.
rajas	Passion; the second of the three gunas (material qualities). It is typified by desire, ambition and creativity. It is often associated with royalty, hence the related term 'raj' (king).
Rama	An incarnation of the Supreme Lord as a perfect righteous king, born as the son of King Dasharatha and his Queen, Kaushalya.
salwar-kameez	Indian women's dress, consisting of tunic, trousers and scarf; this outfit is often worn by women from Punjab.
sampradaya	An unbroken succession of spiritual teachers and their disciples, entrusted to perpetuate a particular philosophy/theology.
samskara	A rite of passage aimed at purifying the soul in its life journey.
Sanatana Dharma	The 'eternal religion' (*see also* dharma); many adherents prefer this to the more recent (and possibly misleading) term 'Hinduism'. It denotes the eternal, dynamic relationship between the individual soul and God.
sannyasi	A man in the sanyassa order, the fourth and final ashram (stage of life). *Sannyasis* take a vow of celibacy, often after married life but sometimes as

	young bachelors wishing to totally avoid marriage. They renounce worldly life.
Sanskrit	The ancient language of the Vedas celebrated for its grammar par excellence. Known as the mother of the Indo-European languages, it is rarely spoken these days, but remains the main language of study and liturgy.
sari	A single piece of cloth worn as traditional dress by many Indian women.
sattva	Goodness; the foremost of the three gunas (material qualities). It is typified by peacefulness, sustainability and wisdom.
sattvic	Imbued with goodness; it is a somewhat anglicised adjective derived from 'sattva'; 'rajasic' and 'tamasic' are similar adjectives.
Shaiva	A follower or worshipper of Lord Shiva.
Shakta	A worshipper of Shakti, the Goddess, also called Durga Kali, Paravati, etc.
shikha	A tuft of hair over the posterior part of the head, often left uncut during the child's head-shaving ceremony.
shraddha	Performance of religious rites after a funeral, such as the scattering of ashes or the offering of sanctified food for all the family's deceased.
shri	A term of respect given to men, male deities and sacred objects, including books; also a name for Lakshmi, the goddess of fortune.
shriman	'Having the favour of the goddess of fortune', an honorific used before the names of gentlemen.
Skanda Purana	A Hindu religious text. The largest of the major 18 *Puranas.*
Swami	Literally 'controller', or more specifically, 'one who can control the senses'. A common term of respect for *sannyasis* and *sadhus* (holy men in general). Alternative forms are 'Swamiji' and 'Goswami'.
Swaminarayan	The founder of the Swaminarayan tradition of Hinduism, one of the main Hindu communities

represented in Britain; is worshipped as God by members of the faith.

tamas	Ignorance; one of the three gunas (material qualities). It is typified by darkness, madness and degradation.
tilak	Auspicious marks of sacred clay and other substances applied daily on the forehead (and sometimes on various limbs as well) to dedicate one's body to God and to denote one's particular religious affiliation.
Trimurti	The three main deities within the Hindu tradition, namely Brahma, Vishnu and Shiva. Each has a respective female consort.
tulasi	A sacred plant, especially worshipped by devotees of Vishnu (often as Krishna or Rama). Tulasi leaves are especially important during Hindu births and deaths.
Upanayana Samskara	Religious initiation ceremony to link the child to God and a lineage of spiritual teachers. Often called 'the sacred thread ceremony'.
upavita	A sacred thread (*see also* janoi).
Vaikuntha	The kingdom of God; literally 'the place of no anxiety'.
Vaishnava	A devotee of Lord Vishnu, or one of his forms such as Krishna.
varna	One of the four occupational divisions in the *varnashrama* social system: the four classifications are *brahmins* (teachers, priests and scholars); *kshatriyas* (rulers, warriors and police); *vaishyas* (traders, farmers and business people); and *shudras* (workers and artisans). Note that it is misleading to call the varnas 'castes'.
varnashrama	The Vedic social system, consisting of four occupational divisions (*varnas*) and four stages of life (*ashramas*). Many Hindus believe that this system, which allowed social mobility, was the forerunner of the current hereditary caste system.

vastu	The Vedic science of architecture and placement; the Indian equivalent of feng shui.
vata	In Ayurvedic medicine, the force or humour symbolised by ether and air.
Vedas	The original Hindu scriptures, which comprise the shruti section of holy books. There are four Vedas. Veda literally means 'knowledge'.
Vedic	Pertaining to the *Vedas*, or more broadly, following or derived from Vedic authority. It also refers to a particular time in the history of Hinduism, marked by veneration of the deities representing nature and the performance of the havana (an ancient fire ceremony).
Vidyarambha Samskara	The ceremony marking the beginning of education.
vipaka	The 'after taste' of food, according to one of several ways of classifying food in the system of Ayurveda.
Vishnuduta	The messengers of Lord Vishnu, said to escort pious souls back to the spiritual world after death.
Vivaha Samskara	Traditional Hindu wedding ceremony.
Yamaraja	The Hindu deity in charge of death and justice.
Yamuna	One of the holiest Hindu rivers. Traditionally, they are seven in number. The Yamuna flows through Vrindavan, the land associated with Krishna.
yoga	Literally means to join. Different yoga systems are described with the ultimate aim of 'union with God'. Upon liberation the soul is reinstated in its original spiritual position: either by merging into the all-pervading brahman (Supreme) or in a personal relationship as the servant of the Lord in the spiritual realm.

As there is no system for capitalization in Sanskrit, we have used lower case even when the translation of the term would warrant a capital letter (e.g. bhagavan, which loosely translates as 'God'). The exceptions are proper names (e.g. Bhagavan Swaminarayan). We have usually used the upper case for Sanatana Dharma as it is often used as an alternative to 'Hinduism'.

Index